Innovative Research in Podiatric Medical Schools

Editor

THOMAS J. CHANG

CLINICS IN PODIATRIC
MEDICINE AND SURGERY

www.podiatric.theclinics.com

Consulting Editor
THOMAS J. CHANG

April 2020 • Volume 37 • Number 2

ELSEVIER

1600 John F. Kennedy Boulevard ● Suite 1800 ● Philadelphia, Pennsylvania, 19103-2899

http://www.theclinics.com

CLINICS IN PODIATRIC MEDICINE AND SURGERY Volume 37, Number 2
April 2020 ISSN 0891-8422, ISBN-13: 978-0-323-73383-0

Editor: Lauren Boyle
Developmental Editor: Nicole Congleton

Clinics in Podiatric Medicine and Surgery (ISSN 0891-8422) is published quarterly by Elsevier Inc., 360 Park Avenue South, New York, NY 10010-1710. Months of issue are January, April, July, and October. Business and Editorial Offices: 1600 John F. Kennedy Blvd., Ste. 1800, Philadelphia, PA 19103-2899. Customer Service Office: 3251 Riverport Lane, Maryland Heights, MO 63043. Periodicals postage paid at New York, NY and additional mailing offices. Subscription prices are $304.00 per year for US individuals, $597.00 per year for US institutions, $100.00 per year for US students and residents, $382.00 per year for Canadian individuals, $721.00 for Canadian institutions, $457.00 for international individuals, $721.00 per year for international institutions, $100.00 per year for Canadian students/residents, and $220.00 per year for foreign students/residents. To receive student/resident rate, orders must be accompanied by name of affiliated institution, date of term, and the *signature* of program/residency coordinator on institution letterhead. Orders will be billed at individual rate until proof of status is received. Foreign air speed delivery is included in all *Clinics* subscription prices. All prices are subject to change without notice. POSTMASTER: Send address changes to *Clinics in Podiatric Medicine and Surgery*, Elsevier Health Sciences Division, Subscription Customer Service, 3251 Riverport Lane, Maryland Heights, MO 63043. **Customer Service: 1-800-654-2452 (US). From outside of the US, call 314-447-8871. Fax: 314-447-8029. E-mail: JournalsCustomerService-usa@elsevier.com (for print support); JournalsOnlineSupport-usa@elsevier.com (for online support).**

Reprints. For copies of 100 or more of articles in this publication, please contact the Commercial Reprints Department, Elsevier Inc., 360 Park Avenue South, New York, NY 10010-1710. Tel.: 212-633-3874; Fax: 212-633-3820; E-mail: reprints@elsevier.com.

Clinics in Podiatric Medicine and Surgery is covered in *MEDLINE/PubMed (Index Medicus) and EMBASE/Excerpta Medica.*

Contributors

EDITOR

THOMAS J. CHANG, DPM
Clinical Professor and Past Chairman, Department of Podiatric Surgery, California College of Podiatric Medicine, Faculty, The Podiatry Institute, Redwood Orthopedic Surgery Associates, Santa Rosa, California, USA

AUTHORS

MEGAN ALLEN, DPM
New Mexico VA Healthcare System, Albuquerque, New Mexico, USA

MARCO AVALOS, MD
Research Associate, Dr. William M. Scholl College of Podiatric Medicine's Center for Lower Extremity Ambulatory Research (CLEAR), North Chicago, Illinois, USA

PETER BARBOSA, PhD
Natural Sciences Department, Universidad del Sagrado Corazón, San Juan, Puerto Rico, USA

JOHN BENNETT, DPM, FACFAS
Associate Professor, College of Podiatric Medicine and Surgery, Des Moines University, Des Moines, Iowa, USA

NICHOLAS PATRICK BLASINGAME, BS
New York College of Podiatric Medicine, New York, New York, USA

ALLAN M. BOIKE, DPM, FACFAS
Dean and CEO, Kent State University College of Podiatric Medicine, Independence, Ohio, USA

TIMOTHY CHEUNG, MS, CPT
DPM-PhD Candidate, School of Graduate and Postdoctoral Studies, Dr. William M. Scholl College of Podiatric Medicine, Rosalind Franklin University of Medicine and Science, North Chicago, Illinois, USA

JAMES C. CONNORS, DPM, FACFAS
Assistant Professor, Division of Surgery and Biomechanics, Kent State University College of Podiatric Medicine, Independence, Ohio, USA

STEVEN COOPERMAN, BS
Podiatric Medical Student, Department of Podiatric Medicine, Surgery, and Biomechanics, Western University College of Podiatric Medicine, Pomona, California, USA

MICHAEL A. COYER, DPM
Private Practice, Orange County Foot and Ankle Surgeon, Irvine, California, USA

RYAN T. CREWS, MS
Assistant Professor, Podiatric Surgery and Applied Biomechanics, Center for Lower Extremity Ambulatory Research (CLEAR), Dr. William M. Scholl College of Podiatric Medicine, Rosalind Franklin University of Medicine and Science, North Chicago, Illinois, USA

JEAN PAUL DARDET
Universidad del Sagrado Corazón, San Juan, Puerto Rico, USA

ERIC DUFFIN, BS
Podiatric Medical Student, Department of Podiatric Medicine, Surgery, and Biomechanics, Western University College of Podiatric Medicine, Pomona, California, USA

TIM DUTRA, DPM, MS, MHCA
Assistant Professor, Biomechanics and Sports Medicine, Clinical Investigator, Department of Applied Biomechanics, California School of Podiatric Medicine, Samuel Merritt University, Oakland, California, USA; Past President, Faculty Org, Samuel Merritt University, 2018-2019, Podiatric Sports Medicine Consultant, Intercollegiate Athletics, University of California, Berkeley, Berkeley, California, USA; Clinical Director, Healthy Athlete Fit Feet Program, Special Olympics, Northern California, Pleasant Hill, California, USA; Board of Directors, Joint Commission on Sports Medicine & Science

ADAM E. FLEISCHER, DPM
Associate Professor, Center for Lower Extremity Ambulatory Research (CLEAR), Dr. William M. Scholl College of Podiatric Medicine, North Chicago, Illinois, USA

MATRONA GIAKOUMIS, DPM, FACFAS
Assistant Professor, Department of Surgical Sciences, New York College of Podiatric Medicine, New York, New York, USA; Faculty, The Podiatry Institute, Decatur, Georgia, USA

CHRISTOPHER GIRGIS, DPM
Center for Lower Extremity Ambulatory Research (CLEAR), Dr. William M. Scholl College of Podiatric Medicine, North Chicago, Illinois, USA

LOGAN GULL, BS
College of Podiatric Medicine and Surgery, Des Moines University, Des Moines, Iowa, USA

ELNAZ HAMEDANI, BA, BS
Podiatric Medical Student, Department of Podiatric Medicine, Surgery, and Biomechanics, Western University College of Podiatric Medicine, Pomona, California, USA

JASON HANFT, DPM, FACFAS
President and Co-Founder, Hansen Pharmaceutical, LLC, Co-Founder, Foot & Ankle Institute of South Florida, Co-Founder, Doctors Research Network, South Miami, Florida, USA

MARK A. HARDY, DPM, FACFAS
Division Head, Division of Surgery and Biomechanics, Kent State University College of Podiatric Medicine, Independence, Ohio, USA

LAWRENCE HARKLESS, DPM
Dean Emeritus, Department of Podiatric Medicine, Surgery, and Biomechanics, Western University College of Podiatric Medicine, Pomona, California, USA

STEPHEN HILL, BSc, MSc, PhD
Adjunct Professor, Podiatry, Physical Therapy, Occupational Therapy, Assistant Professor, Laboratory Manager, Motion Analysis Research Center, Samuel Merritt University, Oakland, California, USA

CHANDLER HUBBARD, DPM
Clinical Instructor, Western University of Health Sciences, Pomona, California, USA; Surgical Resident, Chino Valley Medical Center, Chino, California, USA

JEFFREY JENSEN, DPM, FACFAS
Associate Dean, Program Director, Midwestern University, Professor, Arizona School of Podiatric Medicine, Glendale, Arizona, USA; Co-Founder, Hansen Pharmaceutical, LLC, South Miami, Florida, USA

STEVEN JENSEN, BBA
Vice President, Hansen Pharmaceutical, LLC, South Miami, Florida, USA

MEGAN KINGSTON, BS
College of Podiatric Medicine and Surgery, Des Moines University, Des Moines, Iowa, USA

KRIS KOELEWYN, DPM
2nd Year Resident, Northport VA Medical Center/Stony Brook University Hospital, Northport, New York, USA

KWASI Y. KWAADU, DPM, FACFAS
Associate Professor, Department of Surgery, Temple University School of Podiatric Medicine, Philadelphia, Pennsylvania, USA

JONATHAN LABOVITZ, DPM, FACFAS
Associate Dean, Clinical Education and Graduate Placement, Professor, Western University of Health Sciences, College of Podiatric Medicine, Pomona, California, USA

BRAD LEE PECK, BS
College of Podiatric Medicine and Surgery, Des Moines University, Des Moines, Iowa, USA

LUKE LEFFLER, BS
New York College of Podiatric Medicine, New York, New York, USA

SHELBY McCRAY, MS, RN
Center for Clinical Research, Oakland, California, USA

CHRIS MILLER, PhD, BA, RT
Clinical Consultant, Hansen Pharmaceutical, LLC, South Miami, Florida, USA; Assistant Professor, Faculty of Medicine, Respiratory Division, The University of British Columbia, Vancouver, British Columbia, Canada

RICARDO NAVARRETE, BA, BS
Podiatric Medical Student, Department of Podiatric Medicine, Surgery, and Biomechanics, Western University College of Podiatric Medicine, Pomona, California, USA

DANIEL OKPARE, BS
New York College of Podiatric Medicine, New York, New York, USA

DANIEL PACKERT, MS, HTL
Assistant Professor, Program Director of Histotechnology, College of Nursing and Health Sciences, Barry University, Miami Shores, Florida, USA

GERHILD PACKERT, PhD
Retired, Former Professor, Clinical Biology Department, Barry University, Miami Shores, Florida, USA

NIRAL A. PATEL, MS
DPM Candidate, Dr. William M. Scholl College of Podiatric Medicine, Rosalind Franklin University of Medicine and Science, North Chicago, Illinois, USA

LACEY BETH PECK, DPM
Oregon Foot Care Centers, Hillsboro, Oregon, USA

COLLIN E. PEHDE, DPM, FACFAS
Assistant Professor, College of Podiatric Medicine and Surgery, Des Moines University, Des Moines, Iowa, USA

ALEXANDER M. REYZELMAN, DPM
Professor, Department of Medicine, California School of Podiatric Medicine, Samuel Merritt University, Oakland, California, USA

NOAH J. ROSENBLATT, PhD
Assistant Professor, Center for Lower Extremity Ambulatory Research (CLEAR), Dr. William M. Scholl College of Podiatric Medicine, North Chicago, Illinois, USA

JONATHAN SEUN, BS
Podiatric Medical Student, Department of Podiatric Medicine, Surgery, and Biomechanics, Western University College of Podiatric Medicine, Pomona, California, USA

JARROD SHAPIRO, DPM
Associate Professor, Department of Podiatric Medicine, Surgery, and Biomechanics, Western University College of Podiatric Medicine, Pomona, California, USA

EMILY SHIBATA, BS
Podiatric Medical Student, Department of Podiatric Medicine, Surgery, and Biomechanics, Western University College of Podiatric Medicine, Pomona, California, USA

DAVID SHOFLER, DPM, MSHS
Assistant Professor, Department of Podiatric Medicine, Surgery, and Biomechanics, Western University College of Podiatric Medicine, Pomona, California, USA

ROBERT J. SNYDER, DPM, MSc, CWSP, FFPM RCPS (Glasgow)
Professor and Director of Clinical Research, Barry University School of Podiatric Medicine, Miami Shores, Florida, USA

ROHAN THAMBY, MS
Podiatric Medical Student, Department of Podiatric Medicine, Surgery, and Biomechanics, Western University College of Podiatric Medicine, Pomona, California, USA

STEPHANIE WU, DPM, MS, FACFAS
Dean, Professor, Podiatric Surgery and Applied Biomechanics, Director, Center for Lower Extremity Ambulatory Research (CLEAR), Dr. William M. Scholl College of Podiatric Medicine, Professor, School of Graduate and Postdoctoral Studies, Rosalind Franklin University of Medicine and Science, North Chicago, Illinois, USA

SAI V. YALLA, PhD
Assistant Professor, Podiatric Surgery and Applied Biomechanics, Center for Lower Extremity Ambulatory Research (CLEAR), Dr. William M. Scholl College of Podiatric Medicine, Rosalind Franklin University of Medicine and Science, North Chicago, Illinois, USA

EMILY E. ZULAUF, DPM
Podiatric Surgery Resident, Foot and Ankle Surgery Resident, Grant Medical Center, Columbus, Ohio, USA

Contents

 Video content accompanies this article at http://www.podiatric. theclinics.com.

> This article is a guide to starting a 3-dimensional (3-D) print laboratory; 3-D models of complicated foot and ankle pathology can enhance surgical planning, improve patient and medical trainee education, and aid in research. This article discusses the variables that must be considered when creating a 3-D printing laboratory, including the hardware, software, printing materials, and procedures. Herein is a basic outline of what is required to develop a foot and ankle 3-D printing laboratory.

> Diabetic foot ulcers remain a challenge to practitioners and costly to health care systems. They range from simple to complex and many treatment options are available. By following standard wound care protocols to ensure adequate blood supply, infection control, debridement, wound management, and offloading many diabetic foot ulcers heal in a timely fashion. For those that do not, an underlying foot and ankle musculoskeletal abnormality must be suspected and treated concomitantly with soft tissue treatment. This article presents a systematic orthoplastics approach for surgical treatment of diabetic foot ulcers using the soft tissue reconstructive ladder and the musculoskeletal reconstructive matrix.

> Gaseous nitric oxide under increased atmospheric pressure (gNOp) has shown ability to kill multidrug-resistant bacteria in an in vitro model and in a live mammalian (porcine) model. Factors impacting the kill rate of the multidrug-resistant bacteria include atmospheric pressures, concentration of gaseous NO, flow rate, and duration of application. Using successful in vitro parameters, gNOp showed multilog reduction of bacteria in a live mammalian (porcine) model. The in vitro testing system, using the EpiDerm-FT skin model (stem cell grown skin), was used to develop

Video content accompanies this article at http://www.podiatric. theclinics.com.

Nonunion rate of first metatarsophalangeal joint (MTP) joint arthrodesis is reportedly less than 6%, regardless of fixation type. Robust modern plating constructs aim to decrease incidence of nonunion while also allowing early postoperative weight-bearing. Quicker transition to weight-bearing postoperatively increases patient adherence, decreases adjacent joint stiffness, and reduces risk of deep vein thrombosis in the postoperative period. The purpose of this study was to investigate the effect tibial sesamoid fixation has on first MTP joint arthrodesis.

Direct repair of deep deltoid ruptures after traumatic ankle fracture is not commonly performed. Previous studies overlook the contributions of the medial deltoid to overall ankle stability and long-term patient satisfaction. Historically, deep deltoid injuries have been addressed indirectly through syndesmotic ligament repair. This technique fails to restore, however, the anatomic function of the primary medial stabilizing structure. The oversight of direct deltoid repair may be one contributing factor to the less than optimal outcomes after ankle fractures with syndesmotic injuries. This article reports a positive response with direct deep deltoid repair, at average 5-year follow-up, with 93% positive return to normal function.

Hypovitaminosis D has been established as a global health problem. As an important regulator of skeletal health homeostasis throughout one's life, optimal levels are presumed. Debate, however, still exists surrounding the definition of normal vitamin D levels and what affect hypovitaminosis D has on fracture prevention, fracture healing, and successful arthrodesis. A literature search failed to show any level 1 studies examining hypovitaminosis D and union rates in foot and/or ankle arthrodesis procedures. Several retrospective studies do point to some sort of association between nonunion and hypovitaminosis D. Because of lack of high-level studies, a potential study design is proposed.

A higher incidence of plantar verrucae, commonly known as plantar warts, has been shown in patients infected with the human immunodeficiency virus. Several strains of human papillomavirus are associated with clinical manifestations of plantar verrucae. In this literature review, we examine the incidence and clinical manifestations of plantar verrucae in dual coinfection with human immunodeficiency virus and human papillomavirus. We discuss changes in the clinical scenario brought about by the introduction of human immunodeficiency virus antiretroviral therapy. As a clinical condition with notable presence in podiatric medicine, we also confer these findings to increase clinical awareness with treatment modalities.

VII. Dr. William M. Scholl College of Podiatric Medicine

Noah J. Rosenblatt, Christopher Girgis, Marco Avalos, Adam E. Fleischer, and Ryan T. Crews

Falls present a tremendous challenge to health care systems. This article reviews the literature from the previous 5 years (2014–2019) in terms of methods to assess fall risk and potential steps that can be taken to reduce fall risk for patients visiting podiatric clinics. With regard to assessing fall risk, we discuss the role of a thorough medical history and podiatric assessments of foot problems and deformities that can be performed in the clinic. With regard to fall prevention we consider the role of shoe modification, exercise, pain relief, surgical interventions, and referrals.

Sai V. Yalla, Ryan T. Crews, Niral A. Patel, Timothy Cheung, and Stephanie Wu

Offloading the diabetic foot remains the major consideration for ulceration prevention and healing. This narrative literature review presents a brief overview of current guidelines for offloading the diabetic foot and discusses the implications that come with offloading treatment modalities and their effects on the kinetic chain of the lower extremity. We also present the latest innovative studies from the Dr. William M. Scholl College of Podiatric Medicine at Rosalind Franklin University of Medicine and Science that advance the knowledge in this field and provide avenues for future research opportunities.

VIII. Barry University School of Podiatric Medicine

Robert J. Snyder

Researchers often do not publish negative results; positive outcome reported bias remains rampant. This problem is pervasive throughout the medical continuum. Failure to release less than favorable results could be construed as ethically and morally inappropriate. Failure to make public less than favorable outcomes stifles the scientific process and is contrary to the precepts of the Declaration of Helsinki and the World Health Organization. Sponsors and researchers must embrace the ideal of publishing well-designed studies with negative results.

CLINICS IN PODIATRIC MEDICINE AND SURGERY

FORTHCOMING ISSUES

July 2020
Revisional Surgery
Sean Grambart, *Editor*

October 2020
OrthoplasticTechniques for Lower Extremity Reconstruction
Edgardo R. Rodriguez-Collazo
and Suhail Masadeh, *Editors*

RECENT ISSUES

January 2020
Biomechanics of the Lower Extremity
Jarrod Shapiro, *Editor*

October 2019
Updates in Implants for Foot and Ankle Surgery: 35 Years of Clinical Perspectives
Meagan Jennings, *Editor*

SERIES OF RELATED INTEREST

Foot and Ankle Clinics
Orthopedic Clinics

Foreword

Top Research in the Podiatric Colleges

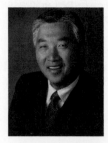

Thomas J. Chang, DPM
Consulting Editor

This issue has been high on my list ever since I took on the role of editor. I was extremely fortunate to start my career in education, teaching within the Department of Podiatric Surgery at the California College of Podiatric Medicine in 1993. It was such a privilege to have participated directly in the education of our students and residents from this grass roots level, and one of the proudest periods of my medical life.

The infrastructure of early success and future growth of our profession will continue to come from the world-class education found within the Colleges of Podiatric Medicine. There is no other medical professional able to provide complete unparalleled care of the foot and ankle and lower leg. This complete training covers all facets of the diabetic foot and wound care, routine palliative care, biomechanical support of the foot and ankle using all forms of orthotic and functional bracing, and complete surgical reconstruction of the foot and ankle. It is only through the educational programs within the podiatric medical schools that the graduates are regarded as the most complete overall providers of foot and ankle care in the world.

It is my hope that all the schools get the attention and recognition they deserve. It is important to acknowledge the commitment of all the faculty members of the podiatric colleges. This issue will serve to highlight some of their research interests and endeavors as they continue to inspire and educate our students.

I am forever grateful to these colleges of podiatric medicine. All nine schools are represented in this Education issue. I hope all practicing and retired podiatrists will continue to remember the tremendous education they were provided and continue

Clin Podiatr Med Surg 37 (2020) xv–xvi
https://doi.org/10.1016/j.cpm.2020.02.001
0891-8422/20/© 2020 Published by Elsevier Inc.

podiatric.theclinics.com

to support these colleges when possible. These schools have given us the foundation of the success we all enjoy in our lives.

Thomas J. Chang, DPM
Redwood Orthopedic Surgery Associates
208 Concourse Boulevard
Santa Rosa, CA 95403, USA

E-mail address:
thomaschang14@comcast.net

I. Des Moines University College of Podiatric Medicine and Surgery

1. Des Moines University College
of Podiatric Medicine and Surgery

Development of a 3-D Printing Laboratory for Foot and Ankle Applications

Collin E. Pehde, DPM*, John Bennett, DPM, Brad Lee Peck, BS, Logan Gull, BS

KEYWORDS

- Foot and ankle 3-D printing • STL • DICOM • Filament • 3-D printer

KEY POINTS

- Foot and ankle models that are 3-dimensional (3-D) printed can be useful for surgical planning, education, and research.
- There are multiple steps required to 3-D print a foot and ankle model from a computed tomography scan.
- There are several factors to consider when selecting a 3-D printer.
- When setting up a 3-D printing laboratory, several factors must be considered including hardware, software, printing materials, and procedures.

Video content accompanies this article at http://www.podiatric.theclinics.com.

INTRODUCTION

Contemporary innovations in 3-dimensional (3-D) printing have resulted in increased usage in the medical field. More economical 3-D printers have made them more widely available, and developments in the materials used allow for easier printing than ever. Perhaps most importantly, the increase in information and resources available online provides medical professionals in almost any setting the ability to create models. Surgeons are using 3-D printing in preoperative planning as well as in patient education. It has been linked to an increase in patient satisfaction, decreased surgery time, and decreased intraoperative x-ray exposure and has even been used to generate bone prosthesis and skin grafts.[1–7] With foot and ankle surgeons often treating complex foot and ankle deformities, the information a 3-D model provides is invaluable. Conventional imaging techniques are used extensively to diagnose and evaluate

College of Podiatric Medicine and Surgery, Des Moines University, 3200 Grand Avenue, Des Moines, IA 50312, USA
* Corresponding author.
E-mail address: Collin.pehde@dmu.edu

Clin Podiatr Med Surg 37 (2020) 195–213
https://doi.org/10.1016/j.cpm.2019.12.011
0891-8422/20/© 2019 Elsevier Inc. All rights reserved.

podiatric.theclinics.com

the severity of pathologies that are present; however, they are limited in that they are 2-dimensional. The ability to produce a 3-D model of a foot and ankle deformity can add insight into complex cases as an additional view to the traditional imaging studies. Several studies have shown the utility of 3-D printed models in planning incisions, performing osteotomies and fusions, and reducing deformities to attain proper alignment of the foot and ankle.[6,8–10] Furthermore, a 3-D model can aid in patient and medical trainee education and enhance foot and ankle research. This article serves as a basic framework of what is required and discusses some of the variables to be considered in starting a 3-D print laboratory. This includes a basic discussion of 3-D printing and considerations that must be made when selecting a 3-D printing machine to produce the models, the software that is used to manipulate the images produced, and the printing materials. Perhaps most important are the processes and challenges faced in converting traditional foot and ankle computed tomography (CT) image studies into a file type that can be used to create a 3-D model.

PRINTING IN 3-DIMENSIONS

Printing in 3-D is a form of additive manufacturing, wherein a digital file is converted to a solid object by converting the file to instructions for a machine that creates the model by adding 1 layer of material on top of another. The way 3-D printers accomplish this varies; 2 of the most popular styles are fused deposition modeling (FDM) and stereolithography (SLA). FDM involves a machine pushing plastic through a nozzle that melts the plastic and deposits it on a print surface as it moves in a programmed pattern. As it moves, it creates layer upon layer of material, forming a model. SLA involves a small vat of liquid resin and using a moving laser to cure the resin as the model bed moves up, away from the liquid, forming layer upon layer of cured resin.[11] The Des Moines

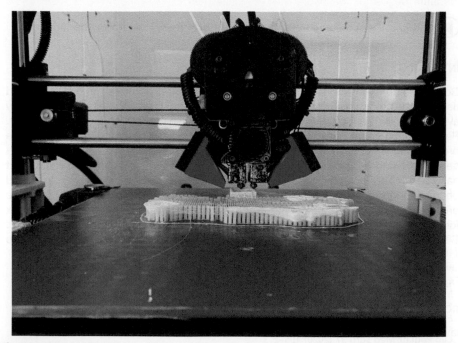

Fig. 1. LulzBot FDM printer with dual-head extruder printing a model. (*Courtesy of* LulzBot, Loveland, CO.)

University (DMU) Foot and Ankle 3D Printing Laboratory utilizes an FDM-style printer and thus is the focus of this article (**Fig. 1**).

THE 3-D PRINTING LABORATORY

When setting up a 3-D printing laboratory, many factors must be taken into consideration.

- Laboratory space
  - Laboratory equipment
  - Storage of models and printing filament
- Laboratory procedures
  - Standard protocols for model processing and printing
  - Postprinting protocols
  - Machine maintenance
  - Laboratory personnel training
- Hardware
  - 3-D printer
  - Computer to process and store models
- Filament
  - Filament dryer
- Software
  - Slicing and model processing
  - 3-D printer program

LABORATORY SPACE

Adequate space for the printer is a requisite; just as important is a temperature-controlled environment. If the build surface of the printer is not enclosed, taking into account any air vents and ductwork is important in protecting the printer from drafts and excessive temperature fluctuations. This helps ensure consistent results in printing. Filament type also must be taken into account. Some filaments, such as acrylonitrile butadiene styrene (ABS), have a strong odor when they are printed. In order to mitigate the fumes, adequate ventilation is necessary. If the workspace is in a shared laboratory, another filament may be a better option.

Counter space also is important when placing the printer, computer, dryer, and any other equipment. The filament is most effective if it is in the dryer and spooled directly into the machine, so preparing enough space to accommodate the dryer and printer to be adjacent is important. It also is necessary to have enough bench space to work on the models after they are printed (**Fig. 2**).

A large enough storage area is needed to accommodate filament; spare parts, such as print heads; model processing tools; and a removable closure. If the CT scans that are printing come in the form of a disc, having locking storage is something to consider and may be required based on an organizations' policies. Storage of the finished models also should be taken into account for space requirements. The authors elect to utilize stands for the models in order to store them easily on shelves (**Figs. 3–5**).

PROCEDURES

Having written procedures in place is vitally important for a laboratory to produce quality, replicable results. This is especially important in a 3-D printing laboratory because there are many steps involved in the process, with many pitfalls. There is

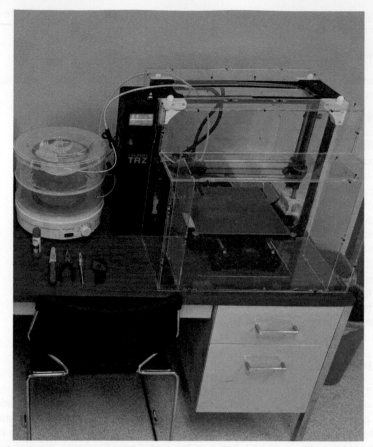

Fig. 2. PrintDry filament dryer and LulzBot TAZ 6 FDM printer. (*Courtesy of* PrintDry™, Windsor, Canada; and LulzBot, Loveland, CO.)

a high learning curve to 3-D printing foot and ankle models; thus, it is essential to have successful processes in place for timely teaching of new laboratory members, to provide a review process for existing team members, and to have continuous quality monitoring. This can be done in a variety of ways, from having someone teach one on one, to going to a workshop, and to self-learning through reading and experimenting. Printing in 3-D is a novel process with scattered information about the necessary techniques. Thus, the authors continue to produce and update the 3-D printing laboratory manual to address the issues of learning, teaching, improving, and maintaining quality prints.

HARDWARE
Printer

The authors have found that an FDM machine has properties that are the most appropriate for the laboratory (**Fig. 6**).

The ability to use multiple types of filament with different properties and colors is important for the authors' models. Being able to utilize dissolvable support material is advantageous to maintaining detail in tight spaces common in foot and ankle models (**Fig. 7**).

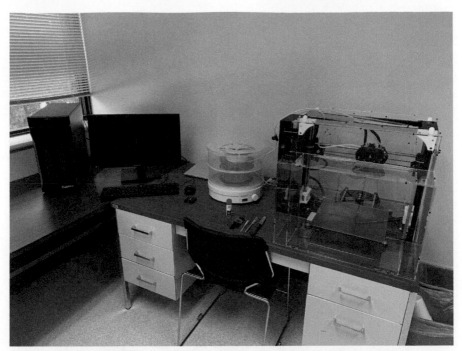

Fig. 3. Laboratory workspace images of LulzBot TAZ 6 and PrintDry. (*Courtesy of* Lulzbot, Loveland, CO; and of PrintDry™, Windsor, Canada.)

The print bed is a vital part of the printer and has several aspects that must be considered when selecting a printer. First is the size of the build area. The size of the models to be produced is determined by the size of the print bed surface, and models must be large enough to appreciate foot and ankle pathology. Larger build volumes correlate with increased prices of 3-D printers. Furthermore, the cost of an FDM printer with a build plate of comparable size to an SLA printer is significantly less. The authors' print bed size is 280 mm × 280 mm × 250 mm.

Second is how the bed is leveled. It is vital that the machine is able to determine where the part that it is producing is in space. Leveling the print bed allows the height of the nozzle to be set and the machine then to be able to predict where the bed will be. This can be a painstaking process and is vital to print success. The authors recommend a printer with a self-leveling bed that utilizes sensors to allow the machine to probe the bed and make a virtual map of the surface. This feature greatly increases efficiency (**Fig. 8**).

A third factor is the bed itself and how well the melted plastic adheres to the print surface. A print must stick to the bed without moving to produce a successful print but also must release with ease at the completion of the print. There are several surfaces that are available and the type of material that is printed plays into this decision. The authors selected a borosilicate glass bed for versatility and great bed adhesion. The print bed also may be heated. This is a feature that greatly enhances the adhesion of some materials and may be necessary for some materials to print successfully.

The printing versatility of the machine is something that also needs to be taken into consideration. Several printers are available with multiple modular print heads that provide different characteristics, such as a dual extruder that allows printing of 2 filaments at once, different-sized nozzles for different levels of precision in a print, and

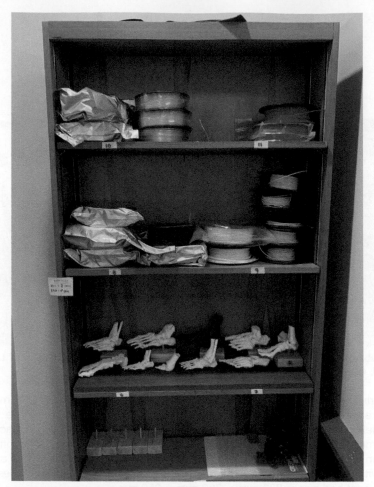

Fig. 4. Laboratory storage for filament and finished models.

others. These modular designs allow the changes to be made in a matter of minutes to facilitate prints of different types (**Figs. 9–12**).

Computer

The desktop computer or laptop computer that is chosen to run a 3-D printing laboratory is crucial to the operation of the projects. All programs have a minimum requirement for both hardware and software to run a program. These requirements are exactly as they are stated, a minimum, and do not necessarily run a program optimally. In addition to this, minimum requirements can change as new versions of the software are released or advances in technology are made. When selecting a computer to purchase, the authors highly recommend working with the information technology department to find the current minimum requirements for the programs to be used and selecting the highest minimum for the baseline in computer selection. Otherwise, the data that are being manipulated can put excessive strain on the computer system, leading to increased load and render times and even program failure. This can make it difficult to troubleshoot issues of poor processing technique of the laboratory worker versus hardware inadequacy.

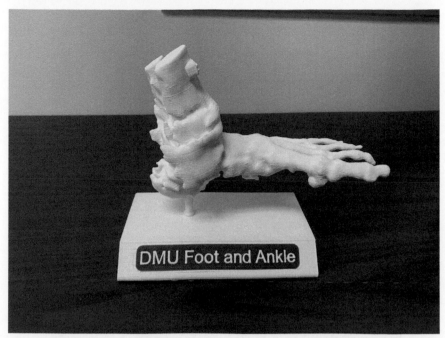

Fig. 5. Completed foot on 3-D printed stand. (*Courtesy of* Des Moines University Foot and Ankle Clinic, Des Moines, IA.)

If making a selection at the time of this article and using the same programs, the current minimum requirements to successfully run the necessary software programs are as follows[12,13]:

- Operating system
  - Windows 7 or newer
  - Mac OS X 10.7 or newer
- Hardware
  - Central processing unit: Intel Core i7 or newer or equivalent (many of the processes that are run are multithread and a multicore configuration is beneficial)
  - Memory: 8 GB
  - Video card: NVIDIA GeForce 580 or equivalent (3-GB GDDR5)
  - Storage: solid-state drive
  - Monitor: 1024 × 768 pixels

To give an example, the program slicer is used to convert a Digital Imaging and Communications in Medicine (DICOM) file to standard tessellation language (STL) and then make edits. DICOM files can come in all sizes. A foot and ankle DICOM can be a few megabytes whereas other files of a spine could be much larger. The performance of the program is directly related to the files size and quality and the tools used to edit or refine these files.

FILAMENT

One of the most important factors in producing a high-quality foot and ankle model is filament selection. FDM printing can use filaments with varying cost and properties.

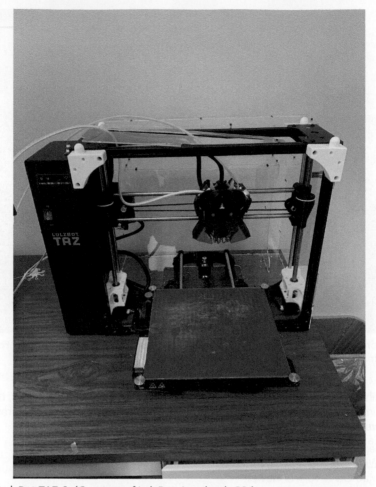

Fig. 6. LulzBot TAZ 6. (*Courtesy of* LulzBot, Loveland, CO.)

The pliability of the material, melting point, ease of printing, and toughness are factors that vary from material to material. The authors have found that the most important consideration is the ease of printing and find that polyacetic acid (PLA) meets the needs. PLA has a relatively low melting point and extrudes through an FDM machine well. It is stiff and resilient enough for a model while being cost-effective. It does not require a heated bed to adhere well and it releases well from the bed when the prints are complete. Polyethylene terephthalate glycol and ABS are other options; however, the authors feel they do not offer the same ease of printing and are less cost-effective.

Polyvinyl alcohol (PVA) is a filament that is dissolvable in water. It can be used in applications where extensive support material is needed, but the scarring from removing the supports is not acceptable. PVA has a similar melting temperature to the PLA filament that is used to create the model. This is vital to getting proper layer adhesion when printing 2 filaments simultaneously. The supports for the authors' models typically dissolve in approximately 4 hours (**Fig. 13**).

Storage of filament in a cool, dry environment is important to control humidity. Many of the filaments are hygroscopic and retain water, which can have a deleterious effect

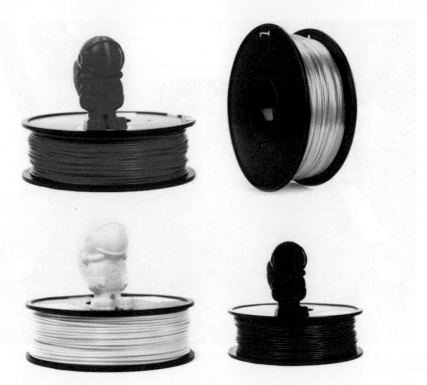

Fig. 7. Matterhackers Filament ([*upper left*] red PLA, [*upper right*] PVA, [*bottom left*] white PLA, and [*bottom right*] blue PLA). (*Courtesy of* MatterHackers, Inc., Foothill Ranch, CA.)

on 3-D model production. The absorbable support material filament the authors use is particularly prone to moisture and needs to be dried and sealed for proper results. To achieve this, the authors utilize a commercial filament dryer with temperature controls (**Fig. 14**). It is large enough to house 2 filament spools at a time and allows the filament to feed directly to the 3-D printer.

SOFTWARE AND COMPUTED TOMOGRAPHY FILE PROCESSING

One of the most challenging aspects of 3-D printing models from CT scan is preparing the file for the 3-D printer to interpret. This requires several steps utilizing multiple software programs. There are many proprietary and open-source options available. At this time, the authors' laboratory utilizes 5 open-source programs (**Fig. 15**).

As a result, there are many new versions and updates available for these programs on a regular basis. The authors have found that updating only when there is a problem that is set to be solved by an update is the best strategy to ensure a continuity of results and allow documentation of procedures to stay up to date. This strategy is utilized universally across all the programs.

DIGITAL IMAGING AND COMMUNICATIONS IN MEDICINE TO STEREOLITHOGRAPHY

The CT scans are delivered in a DICOM file. 3D Slicer is a free open-source program that the authors use to convert the DICOM file into images that can be manipulated and used to create an STL file. STL files are a virtual 3-D mesh model of the images contained in the CT scan. 3D Slicer uses several workspace modules to manipulate

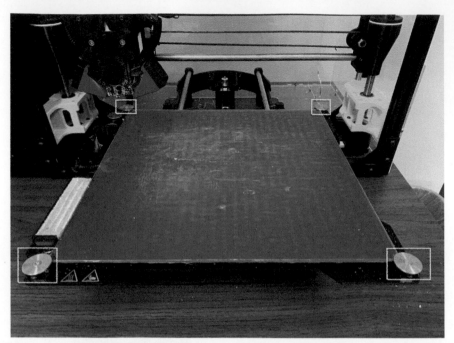

Fig. 8. LulzBot print bed with leveling indicators highlighted. (*Courtesy of* LulzBot, Loveland, CO.)

the files. For instance, the DICOM module is used to select the DICOM file from the computer and pull it into the program. The Segment Editor module is used to select the portion of the CT scan that is used to create the model. The Segment Editor module also contains tools to refine the model, such as the island tool that allows removal

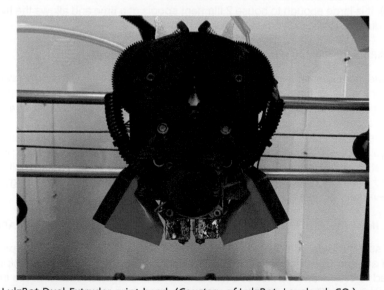

Fig. 9. LulzBot Dual Extruder print head. (*Courtesy of* LulzBot, Loveland, CO.)

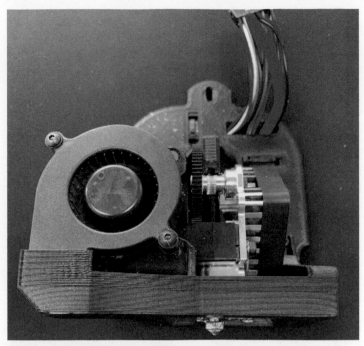

Fig. 10. LulzBot Aerostruder print head. (*Courtesy of* LulzBot, Loveland, CO.)

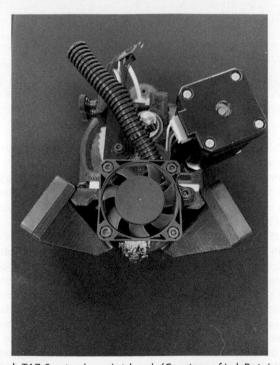

Fig. 11. LulzBotStock TAZ 6 extruder print head. (*Courtesy of* LulzBot, Loveland, CO.)

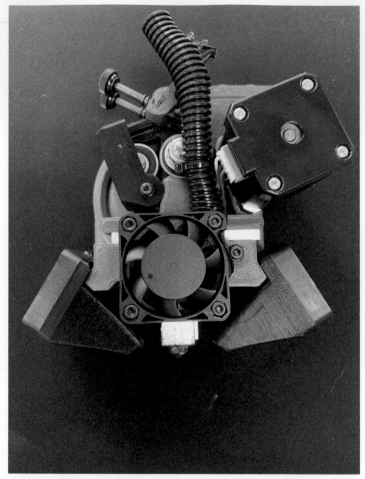

Fig. 12. Lulzbot MOARstruder print head. (*Courtesy of* Lulzbot, Loveland, CO.)

of a cast or boot from the model. The segment that is created is exported as an STL file for further refinement in other programs.

The STL file from 3D Slicer is then loaded into MeshMixer software for further image refinement.[14,15] For example, MeshMixer has a sculpt tool that allows smoothing of any artifacts that may appear from the model creation process. This allows a better finish on the print and a more realistic appearance.

A common problem is that the medulla of the larger bones often is modeled as hollow, particularly in the calcaneus. This extends print time and wastes filament as the printer works to create a model that has these surfaces within the model. Blender is a program that corrects this by creating a new model using only the outer surface of the original.[16–18] This is done by shrinking the outer surface a large sphere to approximate the model as closely as possible. The model that is exported from Blender actually is the sphere that was created and manipulated to duplicate the model.

In order to identify the models, a block with a patient number is created in a computer-aided design software, Fusion 360. A stand for the model is also created in Fusion 360 and 3-D printed. It is subtracted from the calcaneus to create a hole

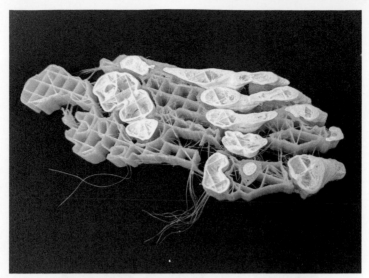

Fig. 13. Partially completed model with PVA (*tan*) and PLA (*white*) filaments.

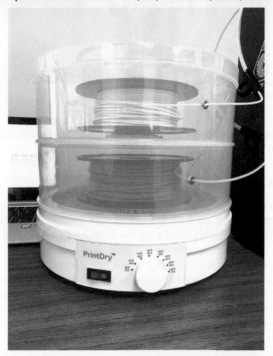

Fig. 14. PrintDry filament dryer. (*Courtesy of* PrintDry™, Windsor, Canada.)

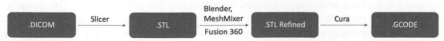

Fig. 15. Process and programs used to take a native CT file (.DICOM) to a printable file (.GCODE).

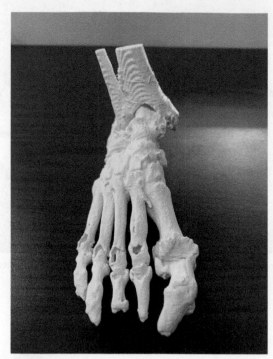

Fig. 16. Rough print of foot.

to mount the model. The models from Fusion 360 are loaded into MeshMixer, where they are combined with the foot model (**Figs. 16–19**).

MODEL CREATION

The final step is to convert the model file into instructions that the 3-D printer can understand. The authors use Cura to accomplish this; these instructions for the printer are a G-code file. The file type is specific for the printer hardware. The print parameters are set within this same software program. This step is different for various printers, and a step-by-step tuning should be performed based on the printer as well as material that is used, prior to attempting to print a model. The settings for the printer are entered, the STL file is imported to the workspace, and the program then is able to slice, or convert, the file. The final instruction set is able to be previewed in Cura to ensure that there are no layers missing or issues with the instructions that are sent to the computer to create the model.

PRINTING AND POSTPROCESSING

Due to the nature of FDM printing, the models must be stuck to the printing surface. The difficulty of removing the prints depends on how well the bed adheres to the material and the surface area that is printed directly onto the build surface. The parameters for the print that are set up in Cura also play a role in part removal from the print surface. The temperature of the initial layer, as well as the layer height, can affect how well the plastic adheres. Care must be taken to not harm the model or the print surface during this step. Sometimes a reasonable amount of force is required to remove the

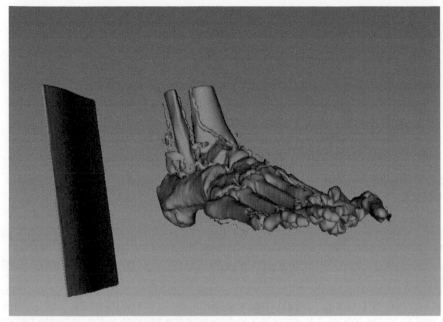

Fig. 17. Rough model of foot in 3D Slicer.

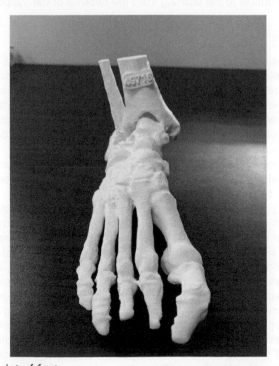

Fig. 18. Refined print of foot.

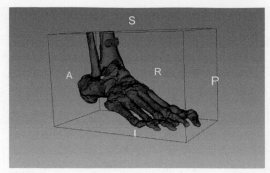

Fig. 19. Refined model of foot in 3D Slicer. A, anterior; I, inferior; P, posterior; R, right; S, superior.

piece. A thin flexible blade often can be used to begin the removal process. This should not require any prying that may damage the print surface or the model.

Most of the models the authors print have overhangs that require supports that must be removed to print properly (Video 1). Many factors regarding the supports are determined by the settings in the G-code that are customizable in Cura or another program that converts STL files to G-code. This support material connects to the print surface as well as to the model. It is important to fine-tune the settings in the software before printing to ensure easy removal of the support material without compromising the model. PVA is a printing filament that is soluble in water. With a dual extruder, this allows printing the model directly on the support material with no gap. When the PVA is dissolved, the model is not susceptible to the scarring from the removal of the support.

CASE STUDY

A 56-year old type 2 diabetic male presented with a left midfoot dislocation with rocker-bottom deformity secondary to Charcot foot trauma that occurred 3 years previously. He was treated nonsurgically, resulting in the foot healing in a malposition. He now has a chronic plantar midfoot ulcer of 1-year duration that is resistant to healing despite comprehensive wound management and offloading. The patient and his wife were seeking an alternative, more permanent treatment solution to address the underlying cause of the ulceration.

The authors discussed surgical reconstructive options to restore a plantigrade, biomechanically stable foot that would allow a heel-to-forefoot gait pattern to prevent inappropriate destructive soft tissue forces.

Weight-bearing radiographs revealed complicated midfoot fracture dislocations with plantar arch osteophyte formation. No signs of foreign body, gas, or deep osseous infection were present. Due to the complex nature of the fracture and dislocation pattern, a simulated weight-bearing CT scan with 3-D reconstruction was performed. The midfoot destructive changes were better understood, especially in the area of the calcaneal–cuboid–fourth and fifth metatarsal base complex, however still a challenge because analysis was still in 2 dimensions. A 3-D printed model based on the CT was printed utilizing the DMU Foot and Ankle 3D Printing Lab.

The 3-D printed model was invaluable to understanding the dislocation pattern, which revealed more accentuated rotation and plantar medial deviation of the calcaneal cuboid joint (not appreciated on the plain radiograph) with significant dorsal, proximal migration of the fourth and fifth metatarsal bases. This allowed more precise preoperative surgical planning for osteotomy placement. This also aided patient education about his complex deformity and the goals of the planned surgical procedures.

The patient underwent reconstructive surgery consisting of gastrocnemius recession to correct the ankle equinus, cuboid dislocation reduction with fusion,

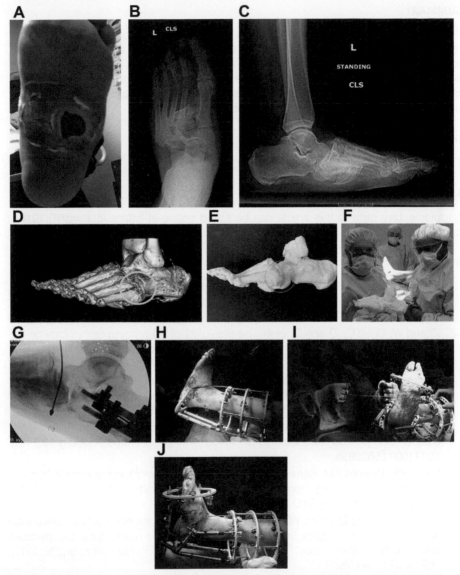

Fig. 20. Preoperative. (*A*) Clinical. (*B*) Radiograph of anteroposterior foot. (*C*) Radiograph of lateral foot. (*D*) CT 3-D reconstruction. Circle denotes significant calcaneocuboid dislocation and fourth to fifth metatarsal cuboid dislocation. (*E*) 3-D printed model shows even further accentuation of calcaneocuboid and fourth to fifth metatarsal cuboid dislocation. (*F*) Intraoperative utilization of model. (*G*) Lateral radiograph with olive wire in place for calcaneocuboid joint arthrodesis. (*H*) Olive wire inferior to calcaneal cuboid joint extended dorsally to inferior tibial external fixator ring. (*I*) Gigli saw midfoot osteotomy. (*J*) Completed reconstruction.

percutaneous midfoot gigli saw osteotomy with reduction of midfoot deformity, and application of Ilizarov circular ring external fixation. The 3-D printed model was useful intraoperatively to help guide reduction and midfoot osteotomy and the authors believe helped cut down on surgical time (**Fig. 20**).

SUMMARY

Foot and ankle models printed in 3-D are proving useful for preoperative planning, research, and patient and trainee education. When setting up a 3-D printing laboratory, many facets must be considered. The space, equipment, printing material, and software are important aspects of the laboratory. The authors have found the learning curve for 3-D printing high-quality models is high but achievable with training and practice following written protocols in a laboratory manual.

DISCLOSURE

The authors have nothing to disclose.

SUPPLEMENTARY DATA

Supplementary data to this article can be found online at https://doi.org/10.1016/j.cpm.2019.12.011.

REFERENCES

1. Cubo N, Garcia M, Del Cañizo JF, et al. 3D bioprinting of functional human skin: production and in vivo analysis. Biofabrication 2017. https://doi.org/10.1088/1758-5090/9/1/015006.

2. Zheng W, Chen C, Zhang C, et al. The feasibility of 3D printing technology on the treatment of pilon fracture and its effect on doctor-patient communication. Biomed Res Int 2018;2018. https://doi.org/10.1155/2018/8054698.

3. Dekker TJ, Steele JR, Federer AE, et al. Use of patient-specific 3D-printed Titanium implants for complex foot and ankle limb salvage, deformity correction, and arthrodesis procedures. Foot Ankle Int 2018;39(8):916–21.

4. Hamid KS, Parekh SG, Adams SB. Salvage of severe foot and ankle trauma with a 3D printed scaffold. Foot Ankle Int 2016. https://doi.org/10.1177/1071100715620895.

5. Smith KE, Dupont KM, Safranski DL, et al. Use of 3D printed bone plate in novel technique to surgically correct hallux valgus deformities. Tech Orthop 2016. https://doi.org/10.1097/BTO.0000000000000189.

6. Chung KJ, Hong DY, Kim YT, et al. Preshaping plates for minimally invasive fixation of calcaneal fractures using a real-size 3D-printed model as a preoperative and intraoperative tool. Foot Ankle Int 2014. https://doi.org/10.1177/1071100714544522.

7. Tracey J, Arora D, Gross CE, et al. Custom 3D-printed total Talar prostheses restore normal joint anatomy throughout the Hindfoot. Foot Ankle Spec 2019;12(1):39–48.

8. Giovinco NA, Dunn SP, Dowling L, et al. A novel combination of printed 3-dimensional anatomic templates and computer-assisted surgical simulation for virtual preoperative planning in charcot foot reconstruction. J Foot Ankle Surg 2012. https://doi.org/10.1053/j.jfas.2012.01.014.

9. Jastifer JR, Gustafson PA. Three-dimensional printing and surgical simulation for preoperative planning of deformity correction in foot and ankle surgery. J Foot Ankle Surg 2017;56(1):191–5.
10. Chae MP, Lin F, Spychal RT, et al. 3D-printed haptic "reverse" models for preoperative planning in soft tissue reconstruction: a case report. Microsurgery 2015. https://doi.org/10.1002/micr.22293.
11. 3d Hubs. What is 3d printing? The definitive guide. Available at: https://www.3dhubs.com/guides/3d-printing/. Accessed September 1, 2019.
12. Ton Roosendaal.Hardware Requirements (Blender 2.80). Available at: https://www.blender.org/download/requirements/. Accessed September 4, 2019.
13. Matterhackers. Makerjuice standard black resin. Available at: https://www.matterhackers.com/store/l/makerjuice-standard-black-resin-1-liter/sk/MJTLHNKZ. Accessed September 4, 2019.
14. Mike Itagaki. 3D printing of bones from CT scans: a tutorial on quickly correcting extensive mesh errors using blender and MeshMixer. Available at: https://www.embodi3d.com/blogs/entry/129-3d-printing-of-bones-from-ct-scans-a-tutorial-on-quickly-correcting-extensive-mesh-errors-using-blender-and-meshmixer/. Accessed September 4, 2019.
15. Pieper S. Recommended hardware configuration (slicer 4.80). Available at: https://www.slicer.org/wiki/Documentation/4.8/SlicerApplication/HardwareConfiguration. Accessed September 4, 2019.
16. lulzbot.com.Cura lulzbot edition hardware requirements (Cura Lulzbot edition 3.6.18). Available at: https://www.lulzbot.com/cura. Accessed September 4, 2019.
17. meshmixer.com.System requirements (MeshMixer 3.5). Available at: http://www.meshmixer.com/download.html. Accessed September 4, 2019.
18. Auto desk knowledge network.Hardware requirements (autodesk fusion 360 2.0.6263). Available at: https://knowledge.autodesk.com/support/fusion-360/troubleshooting/caas/sfdcarticles/sfdcarticles/System-requirements-for-Autodesk-Fusion-360.html. Accessed September 4, 2019.

Orthoplastic Approach for Surgical Treatment of Diabetic Foot Ulcers

Collin E. Pehde, DPM*, John Bennett, DPM, Megan Kingston, BS

KEYWORDS

- Diabetic ulcers • Limb salvage • Orthoplastics • Soft tissue flaps
- Foot and ankle deformity

KEY POINTS

- Diabetic foot and ankle ulcers range from the simple to the complex.
- Successful treatment of diabetic foot and ankle ulcers requires concomitant treatment of musculoskeletal and soft tissue abnormalities.
- Surgical treatment of diabetic foot and ankle ulcers requires mastery of the anatomy of the lower extremity soft tissue envelope and musculoskeletal system.
- Surgical treatment of diabetic foot and ankle ulcers requires a systematic approach using the soft tissue reconstructive ladder and musculoskeletal reconstructive matrix.

INTRODUCTION

Despite advances in medical management coupled with diet and behavior education, diabetes mellitus remains a major health care issue in the United States and worldwide. There is a significant amount of acute and chronic medical conditions associated with diabetes mellitus, which are extremely detrimental to overall health and quality of life.[1] Diabetic foot and ankle complications are one such condition that negatively impact many people. It is estimated that in a single year, 9.1 million to 26.1 million patients with diabetes worldwide develop a foot ulcer.[2] The deleterious impact of a diabetic foot ulcer on a person is significant, commonly leading to partial or complete foot amputation. Mortality caused by a diabetes-related foot amputation can range from 52% to 80% at 5 years.[3]

Over the last several years, the concept of diabetic limb salvage has continued to grow as the need for advanced foot and ankle ulcer treatment has been required to prevent major amputations among patients with diabetes.[4] The goal is to heal diabetic

College of Podiatric Medicine and Surgery, Des Moines University, 3200 Grand Avenue, Des Moines, IA 50312, USA
* Corresponding author.
E-mail address: cepehde@gmail.com

Clin Podiatr Med Surg 37 (2020) 215–230
https://doi.org/10.1016/j.cpm.2019.12.001
0891-8422/20/© 2019 Elsevier Inc. All rights reserved.

foot ulcers in the most efficient and economical manner and provide a stable, functional foot that is not prone to skin breakdown. To achieve this goal, concomitant treatment of ulcers and underlying musculoskeletal abnormalities contributing to increased mechanical stress should be addressed.[5] There are countless treatment options, which can be overwhelming, even for seasoned foot and ankle surgeons. Furthermore, teaching diabetic foot and ankle ulcer management to podiatric medical students, residents, and fellows is a challenge. At Des Moines University, to best guide surgical management of diabetic foot and ankle ulcers and to teach medical students, a systematic orthoplastics approach is used.

DIABETIC ULCER MANAGEMENT

Diabetic foot ulcer treatments range from straightforward to complex, and in many instances requires a team approach from multiple health care specialists for appropriate, efficient management. It is important to institute the basic tenets of diabetic ulcer treatment including[6]

- Infection management with topical, oral, and intravenous antibiotics as necessary
- Optimization of lower extremity arterial inflow and control of lower extremity edema
- Regular, thorough ulcer debridement
- Application of appropriate wound care products
- Nonsurgical foot and ankle offloading
- Management of medical comorbidities

By doing so, many diabetic ulcers heal in a timely fashion. It has been shown that if a diabetic ulcer heals by at least 50% in the first 4 weeks of treatment then there is a high probability of healing by 12 weeks. If not, then there is high a probability that it will not heal and it is recommend more advanced modalities be instituted.[7]

In many instances, lack of healing is caused by underlying foot and ankle musculoskeletal abnormalities coupled with peripheral neuropathy. Common foot deformities, such as bunions, hammertoes, and pes planus, lead to difficult shoe fit, increased plantar pressures, and altered gait in patients with diabetes prone to ulceration.[8]

A thorough physical examination to determine the extent of musculoskeletal abnormality should be performed and standing foot and ankle radiographs to assess the extent of deformity.[9] We have found in complicated deformities that simulated weight-bearing computed tomography (CT) scans with the ankle at 90° with three-dimensional (3D) reconstructions are helpful with surgical planning. The advent of weight-bearing CT scanners is also promising.[10] We have also developed a 3D printing laboratory for foot and ankle models based on CT scans, which have proven invaluable.

Once the ulcer severity is established and the extent of any underlying foot and ankle musculoskeletal abnormality is defined, a surgical treatment plan should be created based on the individual patient. Patient factors to consider include

- Age
- Ambulatory status
- Contralateral partial or complete foot amputation
- Motivation to salvage the foot
- Support network
- Ability to comply with weight-bearing restrictions

- Nutritional status and diabetes control
- Peripheral vascular disease control (arterial and venous)
- Management of medical comorbid conditions

In many instances a more proximal leg amputation may be the best option for the patient. For example, if a patient has not been ambulatory for a long period of time and the rehabilitation potential for standing and walking is minimal, a more proximal amputation should be considered.[5]

If limb salvage is a viable option, then it should be determined if a partial foot amputation or full foot salvage is the best option. Next, regardless of the complexity of the ulcer and any underlying foot and ankle musculoskeletal deformity, a systematic, comprehensive surgical plan should be used. An orthoplastics approach provides such a surgical framework to address the soft tissue and musculoskeletal structures.

ORTHOPLASTICS DEFINITION AND HISTORY

The orthoplastic approach combines the methodologies and strengths of orthopedic and plastic surgery to simultaneously treat bone and soft tissue damage. The reconstruction of bone and concurrent management of soft tissue provides a foundational framework with a nutritional, vascularized envelope to promote optimal healing.[11]

One of the earliest collaborations between orthopedic and plastic surgery was performed by orthopedic surgeon W. Arbuthnot Lane and plastic surgeon Sir Harold Gillies in 1912. Together they advanced plastic surgery by tending to mutilating facial and jaw injuries in the British Plastic Surgery unit at Sidcup during the Great War.[12]

Modern day orthoplastics is used throughout multiple disciplines with the goal of complete bone to soft tissue management. Board certified in plastic and orthopedic surgery, Dr Scott Levin highlights the importance of the soft tissue reconstructive ladder (STRL) in limb salvage. He describes the vital importance of concurrent bone and soft tissue reconstruction to allow optimal repair throughout the entire injury, avoid adverse sequelae of failed implants and/or fixations, decrease incidence of sepsis, and reduce the risk of amputation.[11] Dr Levin's pivotal, contemporary orthoplastic approach is ideal for treating diabetic foot ulcers recalcitrant to standard treatment tenets.

ORTHOPLASTICS APPROACH

The definitive treatment goal for a diabetic foot ulcer is complete healing and correction of contributing musculoskeletal abnormality to achieve a biomechanically stable, plantigrade foot that can be shod with readily available shoes and braces. Orthoplastics provides a methodical treatment approach by combining the STRL and what we have described as the musculoskeletal reconstructive matrix (MRM) (**Fig. 1**).

SOFT TISSUE RECONSTRUCTIVE LADDER

The STRL is a succinct model for managing simple to complex wounds. It is an algorithm that has been used by plastic surgeons for many years to guide closure of various wounds throughout the body, with much literature being published on it over the last several decades. The higher up on the reconstructive ladder, the more complex the procedures and possible morbidity to the patient (**Fig. 2**).

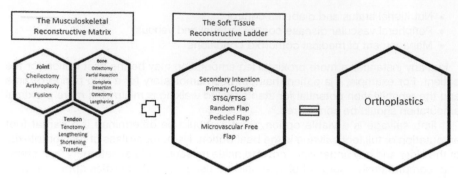

Fig. 1. Orthoplastics model for diabetic limb salvage. FTSG, full-thickness skin graft; STSG, split-thickness skin graft.

Several different variations of the ladder components exist because modifications have been added over the years as treatment options have developed. We have found the STRL is amenable for management of diabetic foot ulcers and have modified the basic ladder to reflect our skill set (**Fig. 3**).

The STRL presents a step-wise approach for surgical wound management, but the clinician is at liberty to skip a step or steps depending on wound circumstances. As an example, the surgeon may elect for a more complex closure method higher on the ladder because of the severity of a wound. The more surgical techniques a practitioner can master, the better equipped to manage diabetic wounds in all stages. To achieve this the surgeon must understand the components of the soft tissue envelope[11,13]:

- Skin: dermis and epidermis
- Subcutaneous tissue
- Fascia
- Muscle
- Periosteum

Several factors must be taken into consideration when choosing the level of the STRL to use when treating a diabetic foot ulcer:

- Where the wound is located
  - Plantar foot versus dorsal foot
- Depth and viability of deep structures of the wound

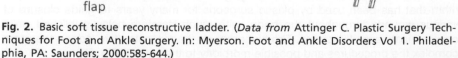

1. Secondary Intention
2. Primary Closure
3. Split thickness or full thickness skin graft
4. Rotation or advancement local random flap
5. Transfer pedicled flap
6. Transfer autogenous microvascular free flap

Fig. 2. Basic soft tissue reconstructive ladder. (*Data from* Attinger C. Plastic Surgery Techniques for Foot and Ankle Surgery. In: Myerson. Foot and Ankle Disorders Vol 1. Philadelphia, PA: Saunders; 2000:585-644.)

DMU Foot and Ankle Approach to the Soft Tissue
Reconstructive Ladder

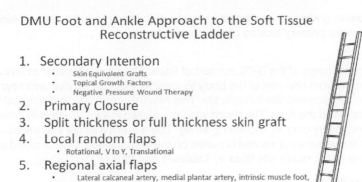

1. Secondary Intention
   - Skin Equivalent Grafts
   - Topical Growth Factors
   - Negative Pressure Wound Therapy

2. Primary Closure

3. Split thickness or full thickness skin graft

4. Local random flaps
   - Rotational, V to Y, Translational

5. Regional axial flaps
   - Lateral calcaneal artery, medial plantar artery, intrinsic muscle foot,
   - Perforator

6. Distant axial flaps
   - Reverse sural artery flap, peroneus brevis, hemisoleus muscle flaps

Fig. 3. The STRL used at Des Moines University foot and ankle. DMU, Des Moines University.

- ○ Bone, tendon, or fascia exposed versus superficial wound
- Acute or chronic deep tissue infection or osteomyelitis

To successfully heal a diabetic foot ulcer, we have found it common to have to move up and down the reconstructive ladder or even be on multiple rungs simultaneously.[11,13,14]

Components of the Soft Tissue Reconstructive Ladder

Secondary intention

This is the first rung of the ladder and the treatment is focused on creating an optimized wound substrate that allows for epithelization. If the wound is chronic or there is exposed bone, cartilage, tendon, or capsule the treatment may be prolonged with standard wound care therapies. It then becomes necessary to use advanced modalities to expedite healing. Over the last several years many advancements have been made including[14]

- Negative pressure wound therapy
- Advanced skin-substitute products
- Topical growth factors
- Wound care dressings for wound optimization

Primary closure

This is the next rung of the ladder and focused on opposing wound edges with suture or staples. It is essential for primary closure the wound is free from infection, has adequate perfusion, and minimal stress on the relaxed skin tension lines.[13]

Split- and full-thickness skin grafts

This is the third rung of the ladder and is useful once the wound bed is optimized and ready to receive a graft. These grafts do not carry their own blood supply and are completely dependent on the perfusion of the recipient site. The two types are

- Split-thickness graft: epidermis with partial dermis
- Full-thickness graft: epidermis with full dermis thickness

We harvest intermediate split-thickness skin grafts at a depth of 0.017 inches with a power dermatome anywhere below the knee. The grafts are typically meshed in a 1:1.5 ratio to allow for larger surface area and to prevent hematoma, seroma, or infection. The harvest site is allowed to heal by secondary intention.[13]

Full-thickness grafts are harvested from the sinus tarsi in a 3:1 ratio of length to width to allow for primary closure of the donor site.[13]

Flaps

The subsequent rungs of the STRL consist of flaps. Flaps are a transfer of tissue with its blood supply from one part of the body to another that can survive until new blood vessels from the recipient site incorporate. This requires more advance surgical skill to raise and then inset the flaps. The donor sites are closed in various ways including primary and secondary closure and skin grafting. There is not a single classification system for soft tissue flaps but instead is based on the composition, type of blood supply, and proximity of the donor site (**Box 1**, **Tables 1** and **2**).[13,15,16]

Local random flaps

These flaps use soft tissue adjacent to the ulcer and are based on a random blood supply. Success is contingent on availability of healthy, pliable, well-vascularized tissue. These are commonly fasciocutaneous flaps and examples include rotational, advancement, and transpositional.[13,15,16]

Regional axial flaps

These flaps use tissue near the soft tissue deficit and are based on a known blood vessel that enters the base of the flap and runs along its axis. Preoperatively, a Doppler is used to map and mark the blood supply to the flap (**Fig. 4**). The flaps are raised as a peninsular (lateral calcaneal artery flap) or island flap (medial plantar artery flap).[13]

Distant axial flaps

The distant axial flap is an island flap that allows transposition of tissue over a larger distance because of the vascular pedicle being dissected from the soft tissues. A Doppler examination preoperatively is imperative to successfully map out the blood supply. To aid in the success in these flaps, especially in higher risk patients, raising the flap and then delaying the inset into the soft tissue deficit by 5 to 7 days is beneficial.[17] Partial loss or wound edge necrosis is a reality and using other components of the STRL may be necessary to complete healing. Examples of these flaps include the reverse sural artery, peroneus brevis, and hemisoleus muscle flaps.[13]

MUSCULOSKELETAL RECONSTRUCTIVE MATRIX

Like the STRL, the MRM serves as a guide for procedure selection to address underlying musculoskeletal abnormalities contributing to lower extremity ulceration. We

---

Box 1
Flap proximity of the donor tissue to the recipient bed

Local
- Use tissue that abuts the soft tissue defect
- Limited by availability of healthy, pliable, well-vascularized tissue

Regional
- Axis flap with a pedicle that used tissue near the defect
- Derive vascular supply from the same anatomic area of the soft tissue defect

Distant
- Flaps using tissue far from the defect and can be transferred over a large distance
- Axis flap with a pedicle or as a free flap

Table 1 Flap composition	
Single Component	**Multiple Component**
Skin	Suprafascial: skin, fat
Muscle	Fasciocutaneous: skin, subcutaneous tissue, fascia
Bone	Musculocutaneous: muscle, fascia, subcutaneous tissue, overlying skin
Fascia	Osteocutaneous: bone, fascia, subcutaneous tissue, overlying skin
	Adiopofascial flap: fat and fascia

came up with the matrix to treat common musculoskeletal conditions that can impede diabetic foot ulcer healing. These include

- Prominent bone
- Bone deformity
- Osteomyelitis
- Joint deformity
- Joint contracture
- Joint instability
- Septic joint
- Tendon and ligament imbalance

The matrix consists of three components with increasing levels of procedure complexity within each. The components include (1) bone, (2) joint, and (3) tendon (**Table 3**).

Bone

Prominent bone coupled with peripheral neuropathy commonly leads to ulceration, especially in the plantar foot. The prominence is caused by native anatomy or aberrance because of fracture malunion, dislocation, or regrowth of osteophytes following partial foot amputations. Bone is manipulated in multiple ways to alleviate these deleterious mechanical forces contributing to foot and ankle ulcers. This includes simplex ostectomy, partial or complete resection of bone segments, osteotomy, or lengthening. It is important to determine if osteomyelitis is present when considering procedure selection. If osteomyelitis is present or highly suspected, a procedure to remove the infected portion of bone should be chosen.

Table 2 Flap blood supply	
Random	Axial
Do not have a specific, named vessel	Based on named blood vessels that enter the base of the flap and runs along its axis
Blood supply is provided by many small unnamed vessels of the subdermal plexus	Peninsular flap contains soft tissue around vessels
Perforator flap	Island flap has a pedicle made up of vascular structures that are dissected from the soft tissue
Base on a perforating artery in which the vessels are dissected out of the tissue through which they perforate	Free flap is detached at the vascular pedicle and must be reanastomosed to artery and vein at recipient site

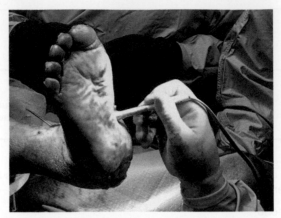

Fig. 4. Using intraoperative Doppler to mark medial plantar artery.

Ostectomy

Ostectomy is a straightforward, useful option for removing undo pressure. The procedure consists of removing underlying prominent bone, with the goal to remove just the amount of bone to be effective. If there is considerable instability of the bone segment or there is concern that removing too much bone may lead to instability, then osteotomy and/or fusion procedures may be warranted instead.[18] For example, plantar midfoot bossing caused by a Charcot rocker-bottom foot is addressed with a simple ostectomy if the prominence is isolated and the midfoot is rigid (**Fig. 5**). If there is instability and/or the ulcer is large, then realignment osteotomy and fusion should be considered.

The calcaneus is a common area of diabetic foot ulceration caused by pressure and friction neuropathic ulcers. A calcaneal gait is also an underlying issue caused by over-lengthening of the posterior muscle group, such as from an overzealous Achilles tendon lengthening procedure or a neglected Achilles tendon rupture. Partial calcanectomies is effective when coupled with appropriate soft tissue coverage for limb salvage.[19]

Bone resection

Partial or complete resection of bone segments is useful, especially when osteomyelitis is present and leading to acute or chronic ulceration. It is important to determine how much stability will be left once the bone segments are removed. If there is concern that the foot and ankle will not be biomechanically stable following resection then a strategy to fill the void may be used.

Table 3		
The musculoskeletal reconstructive matrix		
Bone	**Joint**	**Tendon**
Ostectomy	Cheilectomy	Tenotomy
Partial resection	Arthroplasty	Lengthening
Complete resection	Fusion	Shortening
Osteotomy		Transfer
Lengthening		

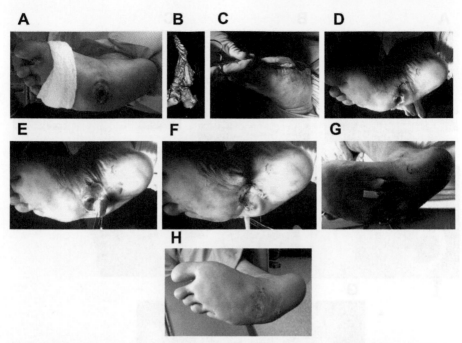

Fig. 5. STRL: random single lobe rotation flap. MRM: fourth metatarsal base ostectomy. Plantar fourth metatarsal base diabetic ulcer secondary to collapse caused by Charcot arthropathy. (*A*) Clinical examination, negative probing to bone. (*B*) 3D reconstruction CT revealing plantar subluxation of fourth metatarsal base. (*C*) Resection of plantar fourth metatarsal base. (*D*) Planning of random local single lobe rotation flap. (*E*) Raising of the flap. (*F*) Inset of the flap. (*G*) Three days postoperative with Penrose drain in place. (*H*) Two months status post-flap.

In the forefoot, plantar metatarsal head ulcers are treated with metatarsal head resections without the need to fill the void. The procedures are especially useful if osteomyelitis is highly suspected or confirmed.[20]

Another common procedure is the removal of tibial and fibular sesamoids for sub first metatarsal head ulcerations (**Fig. 6**).[21] Care should be taken to balance the first metacarpophalangeal joint because of possible dorsal contracture of the extensor hallucis longus tendon. This procedure in many instances is combined with other procedures to resolve plantar first metatarsal head ulcers, such as hallux fusion, metatarsal osteotomy, or tendon transfers.

Partial and complete resection of bone in the midfoot, hindfoot, and ankle region almost always requires a surgical strategy to fill the void or perform an arthrodesis to provide a stable foot (**Fig. 7**). Common strategies include structural bone graft, bone cement spacer, 3D printed cages, or bone lengthening.

Osteotomy

Corrective osteotomies of the foot and ankle are useful to realign osseous segments to reduce undo pressure. They are fixated with internal and external methods or in some cases no fixation is required.

Metatarsal osteotomies are useful to treat plantar forefoot ulcers. The osteotomies are performed proximally, such as a first metatarsal dorsiflexory osteotomy with

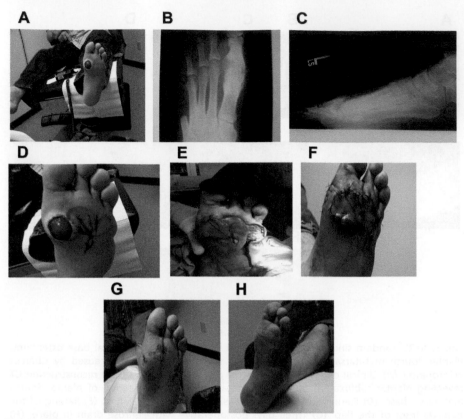

Fig. 6. STRL: local random bilobe rotation flap. MRM: tibial and fibular sesamoidectomy and first metatarsal head ostectomy. (*A*) Clinical examination, first metacarpophalangeal Charcot arthropathy with prominent first metatarsal head and sesamoids. (*B*) Anteroposterior image of foot. (*C*) Lateral foot. (*D*) Preoperative planning for local random bilobe flap. (*E*) Flap raised and inset. (*F*) Five days postoperative. (*G*) Twenty-one days postoperative. (*H*) Nine months postoperative. Note patient has undergone subsequent fourth toe amputation.

fixation.[22] Another useful metatarsal osteotomy is the distal floating osteotomy, which can reestablish uniform plantar forefoot pressures (**Fig. 8**).[23] Midfoot osteotomies are commonly performed in midfoot Charcot deformities to recreate the appropriate calcaneal and forefoot weight-bearing relationship.[24]

Joint

Joint pathology commonly contributes to diabetic ulcerations. This can include limited joint motion, malposition, instability, and infection. Depending on the severity and location of the foot and ankle joint pathology, surgical correction may be required to aid in ulcer healing. The options are either joint-sparing or joint-destructive procedures.

Cheilectomy

Cheilectomy is a joint-sparing procedure that provides increased range of motion of a joint by resecting prominent periarticular bone.[25] This has been a useful procedure to alleviate pressure by increasing first metatarsal phalangeal joint motion for plantar hallux ulcerations secondary to hallux rigidus.

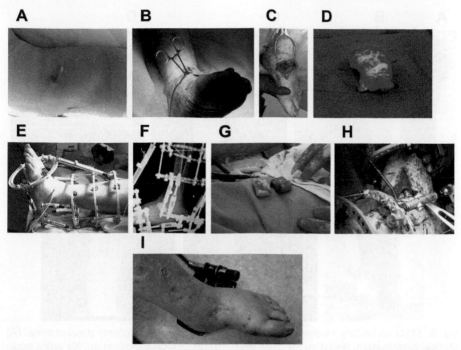

Fig. 7. STRL: primary healing. MRM: resection of navicular with subsequent fusion with allograft. (*A, B*) Diabetic wound following cat bite. (*C, D*) Resection of navicular because of osteomyelitis. (*E, F*) Spanning external fixator to stabilize the medial column with application of polymethyl methacrylate cement bone spacer. (*G*) Tricortical allografts. (*H*) Tricortical allograft application to deficit applied after intravenous antibiotics and serologic evidence of resolving of bone infection. (*I*) Clinical examination 6 months postoperatively.

Arthroplasty

Arthroplasty is a joint-destructive procedure allowing continued joint motion. First metatarsal phalangeal joint arthroplasty has been used for increasing motion to alleviate medial and plantar hallux pressures leading to ulcerations.[26]

Septic joint is also a common cause of nonhealing ulcers. In the forefoot joints, if the distal and proximal osseous and soft tissues are viable, an arthroplasty is a viable treatment option. For example, in a viable toe with an isolated proximal interphalangeal joint ulcer an arthroplasty of the proximal interphalangeal joint can be curative.

Although arthroplasties in the midfoot, hindfoot, and ankle are performed, this may cause too much instability and prevent a functional foot and ankle. Thus, these procedures must be performed with caution.

Fusion

Many diabetic ulcers are caused by joint malposition that is either rigid or flexible. If realignment and stability is required, then fusion of the indicated joints is the best option (**Fig. 9**). If an ulceration has penetrated a joint and there is suspicion or proven septic joint, then fusion may be considered for limb salvage.[27]

Internal and external fixation options are available and dependent on the individual patient case. We typically use external fixation and avoid internal fixation in areas of possible infection.

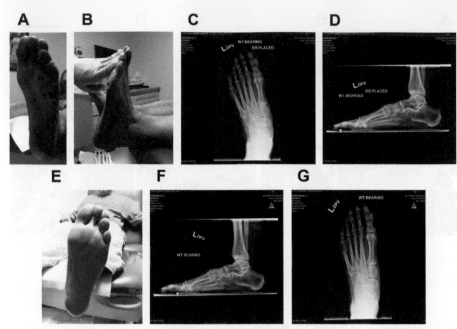

Fig. 8. STRL: secondary healing. MRM: floating metatarsal osteotomy preoperative. (*A*) Clinical examination. Negative for deep probing. (*B*) Clinical examination. No ankle equinus. (*C*) Lateral radiograph. (*D*) Anteroposterior radiograph: marker placed around ulcer 10 months postoperative. (*E*) Fully healed ulcer. (*F*) Lateral radiograph. (*G*) Anteroposterior radiograph.

Tendon

It is common for tendon imbalance about the foot and ankle to lead to ulceration in the patient with neuropathy. To alleviate the aberrant forces the tendon is released through a tenotomy, it is lengthened or shortened, or a transfer is performed.

Tenotomy

Tenotomies are useful for releasing flexion contractures of toes with distal neuropathic ulcers that are free of osteomyelitis (**Fig. 10**).[28] In cases of severe midfoot, hindfoot, and ankle contractures, leading to foot and ankle imbalance, tenotomies are performed. Achilles tenotomy should be done with caution so as not to cause a calcaneal gait that can lead to plantar heel ulcers.

Lengthening

Lengthening overpowering tendons is a useful procedure to reduce pressure. This is done in an open or percutaneous fashion. Probably the most common foot and ankle lengthening procedure is the Achilles tendon lengthening and gastrocnemius recession to alleviate plantar forefoot pressures leading to ulceration.[29]

Transfers

Several foot and ankle tendon transfers have proven useful to redirect and normalize destructive forces leading to ulceration. For the transfers to be effective, the deformities should be mobile and reducible.[30]

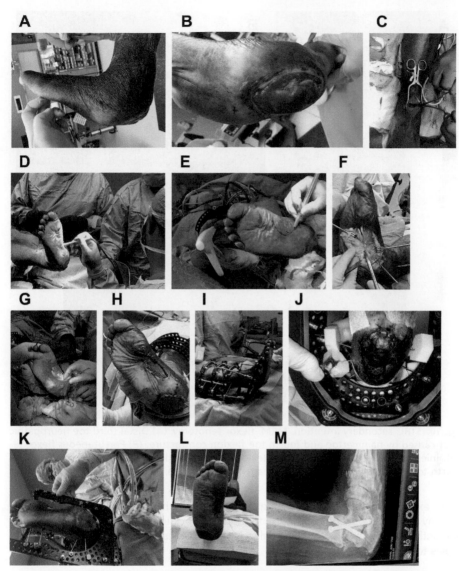

Fig. 9. STRL: medial plantar artery flap, spilt-thickness skin graft. MRM: ankle fusion, partial calcanectomy. (*A*) Excessive dorsiflexion of ankle with calcaneal gait. (*B*) Plantar calcaneal ulcer with hypergranular tissue and exposed bone. (*C*) Ankle fusion. (*D*) Surgical planning with Doppler probe to mark medial plantar artery. (*E*) Marking medial plantar artery flap. (*F*) Raising medial plantar artery flap. (*G*) Flap being inset into heel ulcer. (*H*) Flap sutured in place and medial plantar artery donor site with split-thickness skin graft from calf donor site. (*I*) External fixator used for ankle fusion and to stabilize and offload heel flap (note that external fixator offloading ring is not in place). (*J*) Superficial loss of medial plantar artery flap. (*K*) Debridement of nonviable superficial medial artery plantar flap. Subsequent split-thickness skin graft applied. (*L*) Fourteen months postoperative with fully healed ulcer. (*M*) Radiograph of ankle fusion with internal fixation in place.

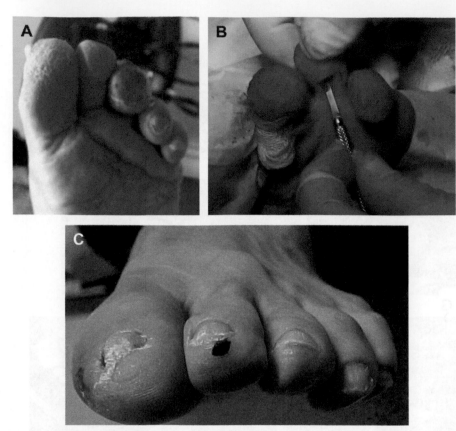

Fig. 10. STRL: secondary intention. MRM: flexor tenotomy. (*A*) Distal third toe neuropathic ulcer caused by hammertoe and fourth toe flexion contracture. (*B*) Percutaneous flexor tenotomies of third and fourth toes. (*C*) Healed third toe with rectus alignment of third and fourth toes. (*Courtesy of* Robert Greenhagen, DPM Omaha, Nebraska.)

For example, in the case of a plantar first metatarsal head ulceration with a flexible first ray Jones tenosuspension is performed to alleviate pressure. If in this case an overactive peroneus longus tendon also is present, it is transferred to the peroneus brevis to also alleviate pressure.[31]

SUMMARY

Management of diabetic foot and ankle ulcers ranges from straightforward to complex, consisting of what seems to be an endless number of treatment options. This inherently creates issues with choosing the appropriate treatments. The goal is to not overtreat or undertreat but to provide the most efficacious treatment based on the individual patient. When a standard diabetic foot ulcer treatment approach is not successful, it is important to assess for underlying musculoskeletal abnormalities and correct with concomitant appropriate soft tissue management. To achieve this, it is imperative the diabetic foot and ankle surgical specialist master the lower extremity anatomy and function of the soft tissue and musculoskeletal systems. This allows a systematic, orthoplastic approach for the surgical treatment of resistant diabetic ulcers using the STRL and MRM.

DISCLOSURE

The authors have nothing to disclose.

REFERENCES

1. United States CDC, National Diabetes Statistics Report, 2017: estimates of diabetes and its burden in the United States 2017: 1–20.
2. Armstrong D, Boulton A, Bus S. Diabetic foot ulcers and their recurrence. N Engl J Med 2017;376:2367–75.
3. Thorud J, Plemmons B, Buckley C, et al. Mortality after nontraumatic major amputation among patients with diabetes and peripheral vascular disease: a systematic review. J Foot Ankle Surg 2016;55:591–9.
4. Driver V, Fabbi M, Lavery L, et al. The costs of diabetic foot: the economic case for the limb salvage team. J Vasc Surg 2010;52:17S–22S.
5. Evans K, Attinger C, Al-Attar A, et al. The importance of limb preservation in the diabetic population. J Diabetes Complications 2011;25:227–31.
6. Amin N, Doupis J. Diabetic foot disease: from the evaluation of the "foot at risk" to the novel diabetic ulcer treatment modalities. World J Diabetes 2016;7:153–64.
7. Sheehan P, Jones P, Caselli A, et al. Percent change in wound area of diabetic foot ulcers over a 4-week period is a robust predictor of complete healing in a 12-week prospective trial. Diabetes Care 2003;26:1879–82.
8. Neville R, Kayssi A, Buescher T, et al. In brief. Curr Probl Surg 2016;53:408–37.
9. Lamm B, Paley D. Deformity correction planning for hindfoot, ankle and lower limb. Clin Podiatr Med Surg 2004;21:305–26.
10. Barg A, Bailey T, Richter M, et al. Weightbearing computed tomography of the foot and ankle: emerging technology topical review. Foot Ankle Int 2018;39: 376–86.
11. Levin SL. The reconstructive ladder: an orthoplastic approach. Orthop Clin North Am 1993;24:393–409.
12. Breakey R, Mulliken J. Sir William Arbuthnot Lane and his contributions to plastic surgery. J Craniofac Surg 2015;26:1504–7.
13. Attinger C. Plastic surgery techniques for foot and ankle surgery. In: Myerson MS, editor. Foot and ankle Disorders, vol. 1. Philadelphia: Saunders; 2000. p. 585–644.
14. Janis J, Attinger C. The new reconstructive ladder: modifications to the traditional model. Plast Reconstr Surg 2011;127:205S–12S.
15. Jeffers L, Basu C. Plastic surgery: essentials for students. Arlington Heights (IL): American Society of Plastic Surgeons; 2012. p. 9–15.
16. Blume P, Donegan R, Schmidt B. The role of plastic surgery for soft tissue coverage of the diabetic foot and ankle. Clin Podiatr Med Surg 2014;31:127–50.
17. Tosun Z, Okkan A, Karacor Z, et al. Delaying the reverse sural artery flap provides predictable results for complicated wound in the diabetic foot. Ann Plast Surg 2005;55:169–73.
18. Catanzariti A, Mendicino R, Haverstock B. Ostectomy for diabetic neuroarthropathy involving the midfoot. J Foot Ankle Surg 2000;39:291–300.
19. Elmarsafi T, Pierre A, Wang K, et al. The vertical contour calcanectomy: an alternative surgical technique to the conventional partial calcanectomy. J Foot Ankle Surg 2019;58:381–6.
20. Faglia E, Clerici G, Caminiti M, et al. Feasibility and effectiveness of internal pedal amputation of phalanx or metatarsal head in diabetic patients with forefoot osteomyelitis. J Foot Ankle Surg 2012;51:593–8.

21. Giurini J, Rosenblum B. Surgical treatment of the diabetic foot. In: Banks A, Downey MS, Martin DE, et al, editors. McGlamry's comprehensive textbook of foot and ankle surgery, vol. 1, 3rd edition. Philadelphia: Lippincott Williams & Wilkins; 2001. p. 1595–616.
22. Pirozzi K, Meyr A. Using geometry for the dorsiflexory wedge osteotomy of the first metatarsal. J Foot Ankle Surg 2014;53:295–7.
23. Tamir E, Finestone A, Avisar E, et al. Mini-Invasive floating metatarsal osteotomy for resistant or recurrent neuropathic plantar metatarsal head ulcers. J Orthop Surg Res 2016;11:1–6.
24. Pinzur M, Schiff A. Deformity and clinical outcomes following operative correction of Charcot foot: a new classification with implications for treatment. Foot Ankle Int 2018;39:265–70.
25. Nicolosi N, Hehemann C, Connors J. Long term follow-up of the cheilectomy for degenerative joint disease of the first metatarsophalangeal joint. J Foot Ankle Surg 2015;54:1010–20.
26. Armstrong D, Lavery L, Vazquez J, et al. Clinical efficacy of the first metatarsophalangel joint arthroplasty as a curative procedure for hallux interphalangeal joint wounds in patients with diabetes. Diabetes Care 2003;26:3284–7.
27. Saltzman C. Salvage of diffuse ankle osteomyelitis by single-stage resection and circumferential frame compression arthrodesis. Iowa Orthop J 2005;25:47–52.
28. Labortde JM. Neuropathic toe ulcers treated with toe flexor tenotomies. Foot Ankle Int 2007;28:1160–4.
29. Greenhagen R, Johnson A, Peterson M, et al. Gastrocnemius recession as an alternative to tendoachillis lengthening for relief of forefoot pressure in a patient with peripheral neuropathy: a case report and description of a technical modification. J Foot Ankle Surg 2010;49:159.e9-13.
30. Miller S, Groves M. Principles of muscle-tendon surgery and tendon transfers. In: Banks A, et al, editors. McGlamry's comprehensive textbook of foot and ankle surgery, vol. 1, 3rd edition. Philadelphia: Lippincott Williams & Wilkins; 2001. p. 1523–66.
31. DiDomenico L, AbdelFattah S, Hassan M. Emerging concepts with tendon transfers. Podiatry Today 2018;31:26–32.

II. Arizona School of Podiatric Medicine

Discovery and Development of Gaseous Nitric Oxide Under Increased Atmospheric Pressure as an Antimicrobial

In Vitro and In Vivo Testing of Nitric Oxide Against Multidrug-Resistant Organisms

Jeffrey Jensen, DPM[a,b,*], Daniel Packert, MS, HTL[c],
Chris Miller, PhD, BA, RT[b,d], Gerhild Packert, PhD[e,1],
Jason Hanft, DPM[b,f,g], Steven Jensen, BBA[b,2]

KEYWORDS

- Nitric oxide • Pressure • Antimicrobial • Infection • Wounds
- Antibiotic-resistant bacteria • Multidrug-resistant bacteria

KEY POINTS

- Gaseous nitric oxide under increased atmospheric pressure has shown the ability to kill multidrug-resistant bacteria in an in vitro model.
- Increasing the concentration of the gaseous nitric oxide reduced the testing time needed to kill multidrug-resistant bacteria in the in vivo model.
- Using successful in vitro parameters, gaseous nitric oxide under increased atmospheric pressure showed multilog reduction of bacteria in a live mammalian (pig) model.
- Delivering gaseous nitric oxide while increasing the pressure at the wound site, and maintaining an appropriate flow of NO gas, shows promising antimicrobial capabilities that should be studied further.

[a] Midwestern University, Arizona School of Podiatric Medicine, 19555 North 59th Avenue, Glendale, AZ 85308, USA; [b] Hansen Pharmaceutical, LLC, 7000 SW 62nd Avenue, Suite 405, South Miami, FL 33143, USA; [c] College of Nursing and Health Sciences, Barry University, Sienna Building, Room 221, 11300 Northeast 2nd Avenue, Miami Shores, FL 33161, USA; [d] Faculty of Medicine, Respiratory Division, The University of British Columbia, Room 258, 2260 Oak Street, Vancouver, British Columbia v5Z 1M9, Canada; [e] Clinical Biology Department, Barry University, 11300 NE 2nd Avenue, Miami Shores, FL 33161, USA; [f] Foot & Ankle Institute of South Florida, 7000 Southwest 62nd Avenue, Suite 405, South Miami, FL 33143, USA; [g] Doctors Research Network, South Miami, FL, USA
[1] Present address: 1343 Southwest 181 Avenue, Pembroke Pines, FL 33029.
[2] Present address: 49 Marion Street, 5D, Brookline, MA 02446.
* Corresponding author. Midwestern University, Arizona School of Podiatric Medicine, 19555 North 59th Avenue, Glendale, AZ 85308.
E-mail address: jjense1@midwestern.edu

Clin Podiatr Med Surg 37 (2020) 231–246
https://doi.org/10.1016/j.cpm.2019.11.001
0891-8422/20/© 2019 Elsevier Inc. All rights reserved.

INTRODUCTION
Wound Healing and Infection

It has been well established that in acute and chronic wounds microbial contamination and infection play significant roles in delaying or preventing wound healing. In fact, it is infection that is the leading cause of wound deterioration, leading to hospital stays, surgical treatment, and in many cases, lower-limb amputation.[1] Diabetic foot ulcerations (DFUs) and subsequent infection are a significant source of morbidity with the potential of limb loss and mortality. The lifetime risk of foot ulceration in patients with diabetes is 15% to 20%.[2] The significant problem in chronic wounds, specifically DFUs, is the lack of consistent healing. Less than 25% of DFUs heal within 12 weeks.[3] If these wounds remain open for extended periods of time, they are more susceptible to infection. Hence, more than half of all DFUs become infected, and 20% of those infected DFUs end in amputation.[4] Sadly, after years of decline, the rate of amputations increased by 50% between 2009 and 2015 to 4.6 for every 1000 adults.[5]

To put this in perspective, the United States sees more than 80,000 lower-extremity amputations to Medicare beneficiaries annually.[6] That number does not take into account the many such procedures that occur on the patient population under 65+ years of age in the United States. The total number is well over 100,000 amputations each year.[5] This problem is a worldwide problem as well, with the World Health Organization acknowledging the diabetic foot complications issue stating, "One lower limb is lost to diabetes every 30 seconds [worldwide]."[7] This situation continues to worsen in large part because specific diseases, such as diabetes, show a dramatic increase in prevalence with projections increasing.[8,9] Currently, diabetes affects more than 30 million individuals in the United States and more than 425 million people worldwide with those numbers projected to increase to more than 40 million and more than 629 million, respectively, by 2045.[8]

Economic Cost

In 2018, *Value in Health* published an article examining the economic impact of chronic nonhealing wounds. The investigators discovered that nearly 15% of US Medicare beneficiaries were diagnosed with a wound or wound infection based on 2014 data. Approximately $98 billion was spent on wound care across the board. In terms of infection-specific spending, this totaled ~$29 billion. Diabetic foot infection–related spending was nearly half of the total infection spending at ~$14 billion.[10] Once again, it should be emphasized that these numbers do not account for the non-Medicare population, so the real scope of this epidemic is even greater.

In a surprising statistic, costs of diabetic foot care and its related limb complications are higher than even the most costly form of cancer in the United States, breast cancer.[11] Of all the insurance costs related to DFUs, nearly two-thirds are inpatient care related.[12] In the cases of patients undergoing amputation, the 2-year costs associated with initial hospitalization, rehospitalizations, postacute care, and prosthesis-related costs were more than $90,000. These patients with amputations additionally face lifetime health care costs projected at more than $500,000.[13] Importantly, this is just the United States alone. Costs related to DFUs are similar throughout the world and are expensive regardless of the health care system.[14] It is important to note that infection precedes amputation in at least 75% of the cases.[4,15,16]

Resistant Infection

Many of the bacteria species that infect wounds have developed resistance to antimicrobial agents. In recent years, bacterial resistance to systemic antibiotics has increased despite the formation of new and improved drugs to help reduce infection.[2,9] Bacterial infections showing antibiotic resistance more than doubled from 2002 to 2014 from 5.2% to 11.0% and result in cost of infection treatment increasing by 165% when facing antibiotic resistance.[17] More than 2 million people suffer antibiotic-resistant infections annually.[18]

The antibiotic-resistant bacteria tested with gaseous nitric oxide under increased atmospheric pressure (gNOp) were the following: *Acinetobacter baumannii*, *Pseudomonas aeruginosa*, *Staphylococcus aureus*, and methicillin-resistant *S aureus* (MRSA). As of 2019, the Centers for Disease Control and Prevention (CDC) have classified *A baumannii* as threat level: urgent; *P aeruginosa* and MRSA classified as threat level: serious; and *S aureus* classified as threat level: concerning. It should be noted that *Staphylococcus* bacteria are a common cause of health care-associated infections. There are more than 400,000 MRSA infections per year leading to more than 10,000 deaths and costing an estimated $1.7 billion annually. *P aeruginosa* is identified in more than 32,000 infections per year. The CDC states that "some types of multidrug-resistant *P. Aeruginosa are resistant to nearly all antibiotics, including carbapenems." A baumannii* infections are fewer in number annually than the previously discussed bacteria; however, *A. baumannii* is "resistant to nearly all antibiotics and few new drugs are in development."[19] The US Department of Defense identified these 4 bacteria as the pathogens to study to evaluate the antimicrobial potential of gaseous nitric oxide (NO) under pressure. Each of these bacteria can be found in diabetic foot ulcers.[20] Therefore, eradicating these pathogens that contribute to the epidemic of chronic, infected wounds is integral to achieving successful outcomes in wound healing in addition to developing new ways of attacking multidrug-resistant organisms. This set of studies evaluates NO as a potential solution to resistant infection in wounds. NO has antimicrobial properties along with numerous wound-healing properties, such as enhancing blood supply, increasing fibroblastic activity, and serving as a potent vasodilator.[21–28]

Nitric Oxide as an Antimicrobial

Gaseous NO is a universal antimicrobial.[21–28] The bactericidal properties of gaseous NO are even more exciting when coupled with avoiding resistance issues. It is unlikely that the infecting organisms develop bacterial resistance against exogenous NO owing to "the multiple mechanisms by which NO presents toxicity toward microbes." Privett and colleagues[23] identify NO's small molecule size and hydrophobicity as key to moving through "bacterial lipid membranes where a number of nitrosative and oxidative reactions may occur," killing the pathogen. Dr Chris Miller and his team have studied the antimicrobial properties of NO since 2004 and have demonstrated that NO, delivered topically, is an effective nonspecific antimicrobial agent against a broad range of microorganisms, gram-positive, gram-negative, and multidrug-resistant strains of bacteria, yeast, viruses, and mycobacteria with no evidence of resistance development.[21,22,28,29] Gaseous NO is thus an exciting potential topical antimicrobial.

One main concern regarding topical antimicrobials is their ability to penetrate tissues to resolve infection within granulation tissue and subcutaneously. The authors' hypothesis for the initial study of gNOp, conducted through a Defense Advanced

Research Projects Agency (DARPA) grant proposal, was that additional atmospheric pressure is needed to allow the gaseous NO to penetrate tissue.

The development of gNOp is reviewed from beginning in vitro testing, through optimization of therapeutic parameters, to an initial in vivo mammalian (porcine) wound testing model. In the initial study, an in vitro testing system was developed using the EpiDerm-FT full-thickness skin model (EFT400), a stem cell grown skin created by MatTek Corporation (Ashland, MA, USA). This tissue was used to develop an infected wound model for the 4 bacteria strains: *A baumannii*, *P aeruginosa*, *S aureus*, and MRSA. A custom-built testing system was developed to control pressure and gas flow inside of a modified Franz cell apparatus. This system was used for all in vitro testing whereby the therapeutic parameters of NO concentration, pressure, gas flow, and time were evaluated and optimized. An in vivo mammalian (porcine) wound model was then developed by Bridge PTS, Inc (San Antonio, TX, USA) to test gNOp against gram-positive and gram-negative bacteria, *S aureus* and *Pseudomonas*, respectively. A partial-thickness wound model, through the dermis but not through the facial layer, was used to mimic diabetic foot wounds. Results were evaluated using colony forming units (CFUs) and respective log-reduction comparing control samples to tested samples.

MATERIALS AND METHODS
In Vitro Testing

Tissue culturing
MatTek EFT-400 skin cultures were obtained from MatTek Corporation. Upon receipt, the tissues were immediately taken out of the growth agar and placed in new sterile 6-well plates. About 2 mL of fresh culture media in liquid form was placed below the tissue inserts, and the tissue was left to stabilize for 24 hours in an incubator set to 37°C and 5% CO_2. Every 24 hours, culture media were replaced to ensure growth of the MatTek EFT400 tissues. The tissue was ready for experiments after the initial 24-hour stabilization period.

Infection assay and growth curves
The in vitro studies used 4 bacteria common with infections and amputations: *A baumannii* (ATCC #BAA-747), *P aeruginosa* (ATCC #BAA-47), *S aureus* (ATCC #12600), and MRSA (ATCC #33591). All work was performed on MatTek epidermal full-thickness skin tissues (EFT-400). Growth curves were established for all bacterial strains in order to develop parameters for the tissue infection model. The final parameters for infection were 15 µL of bacterial suspension grown to optical density (OD) of 1 (10^8 CFU). A single colony of bacteria was isolated from a nutrient agar plate and placed into 4 mL autoclaved nutrient broth. The bacteria-laden broth was then placed on a Thermo Scientific MaxQ 4450 incubated shaker for 18 hours at 37°C and 200 rpm and allowed to grow. After the initial 4 hours on the shaker, 200 µL of this growth was then transferred to 20 mL of fresh nutrient broth and allowed to continue growth for 4 hours at 37°C and 200 rpm. After this latest growth phase, the bacteria were collected and diluted, and the OD was read with a SpectraMax 384 PLUS to obtain an OD600 of 1.00. A 3-mm punch biopsy on the MatTek EFT-400 was made, and 15 µL of the bacteria suspension was used to inoculate the tissue wound and allowed to grow for 24 hours.

Exposure setups with nitric oxide
Infected tissues were set up in modified Franz cell exposure chambers with a custom-built manifold, as seen in **Fig. 1**, capable of adjusting pressure, flow,

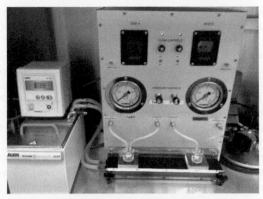

Fig. 1. Manifold for NO delivery, flow adjusted to 100 cc/min.

and length of exposure with gaseous NO. Exposure chambers custom made for the tissue inserts, as seen in **Fig. 2**, were fabricated and used to seal the tissue with the gas. Gaseous NO was then delivered to the exposure chamber from the gas canister, through the manifold. As flow is maintained and pressure is held stable, gas exits the chamber and returns through the manifold to an exhaust system.

In the initial DARPA study, it was determined that a flow rate of 100 cc/min (0.1 L/min) was required for effective use of gaseous NO in vitro. Higher flow rates did not change results; however, lower flow rates did not achieve bacterial kill. Flow is important to maintain a constant new amount of NO gas so that there is

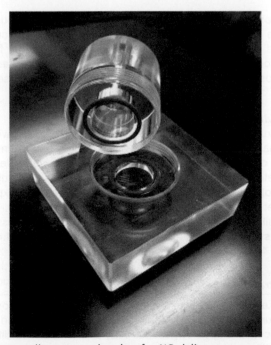

Fig. 2. Modified Franz cell exposure chamber for NO delivery.

no conversion of NO to NO_2, which is both toxic and ineffective as an antimicrobial. Hence, all testing moving forward was completed with a 100 cc/min (0.1 L/min) flow rate.

In the DARPA testing, 1% (10,000 ppm) gaseous NO was floated over the tissue for 90 minutes of exposure against S aureus. Pressure was added and set to 14.7 psi (1 atm) for this duration. These parameters were compared with air at no pressure, air under 14.7 psi (1 atm), and 1% gaseous NO at no pressure. Then, 1% gaseous NO under pressure at 14.7 psi (atm) was tested against the remaining bacteria wound models. Each experiment was run 3 times, with a total of 3 infected tissues each for a total of 9 treated infected tissue models.

The next set of in vitro testing was conducted to evaluate whether lower pressures could achieve a similar result. S aureus had previously proved the most difficult pathogen to kill, so it was selected for evaluation at 4.4 psi (0.3 atm) and 3.7 psi (0.25 atm). Concentration, flow, and time were all held constant at 1% gaseous NO, 100 cc/min, and 90 minutes, respectively.

Once understood that lower pressures could maintain an antimicrobial effect with gaseous NO, a new goal of lowering procedure time was adapted. In order to achieve a lower time, it was hypothesized that an increase in concentration of the gaseous NO might achieve that intended result. This testing primarily evaluated the following parameters: 2% (20,000 ppm) gaseous NO, a flow rate of 100 cc/min (0.1 L/min), pressure of 3.7 psi (0.25 atm), and an exposure time of 40 minutes. This testing evaluated these parameters against all 4 bacteria strains. After these studies, NO above atmospheric pressure was then referred to as gNOp.

In Vivo Testing: Mammalian (Porcine) Model

Infection assay
Infections were completed at Bridge PTS using their approved wound infection protocols for porcine experimental subjects. This infection included creating a partial-thickness wound, through the dermis but not through the fascial layer, to mimic typical diabetic foot wounds, infecting the wounds with S aureus and P aeruginosa (Gram positive and Gram negative, respectively) for subsequent exposure to gNOp.

Exposure setup with nitric oxide
Fabricated exposure devices made of material nonreactive to NO were developed to hold this additional pressure at the wound site for the required time, while the 2% gaseous NO was delivered to the wound interface via a custom-designed manifold. Exposure parameters were set up on this manifold capable of adjusting pressure, flow, and length of exposure with 2% gaseous NO. During the exposure of gNOp, flow rates were set to 100 cc/min (0.1 L/min) for all the experiments. To test the effectiveness of the multiple parameters, testing included varying the pressure and the time of exposure. This study primarily focused on 3.7psi (0.25 atm) and 4.4 psi (0.3 atm) for timed intervals of 40 and 50 minutes.

Thiazolyl Blue Tetrazolium Bromide Tissue Viability

During the in vivo experiments, thiazolyl blue tetrazolium bromide, or methylthiazolyl-diphenyl-tetrazolium bromide (MTT), viability assays were conducted to assess the effect of pressure, concentration of gaseous NO, and time on viability of the MatTek tissue and the healthy porcine tissue.

Histologic Samples

Histologic samples were taken during the in vivo mammalian wound model to assess the effect of gNOp on the wounded and healthy porcine tissue.

RESULTS AND DISCUSSION
In Vitro Testing

Initial Defense Advanced Research Projects Agency proof of concept study

The results of the DARPA study experiments showed a clear indication that gNOp has a powerful time, pressure, and concentration antimicrobial effect. **Fig. 3** demonstrates that although the gaseous NO itself has an antimicrobial effect, the addition of pressure enhances this property drastically. **Fig. 3** also shows that pressure alone with the presence of air has no desirable effect on the bacteria load: the gaseous NO is a necessity.

The results also show a reduction in bacteria after gNOp treatment of the different species. **Fig. 4** indicates the bacteria reduction versus a nontreated control (without pressure or gaseous NO) after 90 minutes of exposure with gNOp at 14.7 psi (1 atm) of pressure. The effectiveness of the gNOp treatment between both gram-positive and gram-negative bacteria was similar in this study. The S aureus (ATCC #12600) is a biofilm-forming strain that proved the most difficult to eradicate with gNOp exposure. Thus, S aureus was selected as the infection control model to determine the specific ranges for the experimental design. These results demonstrate NO's ability to universally eradicate bacteria, whether Gram positive or Gram negative. Based on these in vitro studies, gNOp has significant potential in wound care applications given most infections are not single species.

Next, regarding the MTT assays, the results in **Fig. 5** demonstrate that tissue viability is not affected by the infection itself (columns 3–6) when compared with wounded only and noninfected tissues (columns 1 and 2). Pressure itself also does not meaningfully affect viability (columns 7 and 8). The combination of pressure and NO concentration however is significant. There is a large decrease in viability as NO concentration increases, first without pressure (columns 11, 13), and even more greater with added pressure (column 12 1% NO, +1 atm pressure). In addition, gaseous NO concentration levels are also significant, and the higher the concentration (10,000–20,000 parts per million), the greater the decrease in viability. As

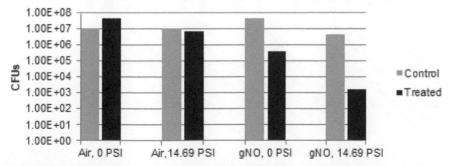

Fig. 3. Determine significance of pressure with and without gaseous NO on reduction of bioburden. 24-hour infection, 90 minutes; 0 or +14.69 psi, flow 0.1 L/min, pathogen S aureus. Control = infected, untreated tissue, 3 sets of triplicates per experiment.

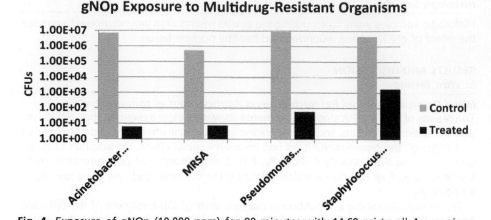

Fig. 4. Exposure of gNOp (10,000 ppm) for 90 minutes with 14.69 psi to all 4 organisms ($\log_{10}$ CFU/g).

exposure time is decreased, viability increases in the presence of 1% NO with or without pressure (columns 13–16). An important factor to consider in relating the in vitro model to an in vivo model is the fact that the tissue has no way of breaking down the gaseous NO by-products (nitrites and nitrates) that cells in a living system

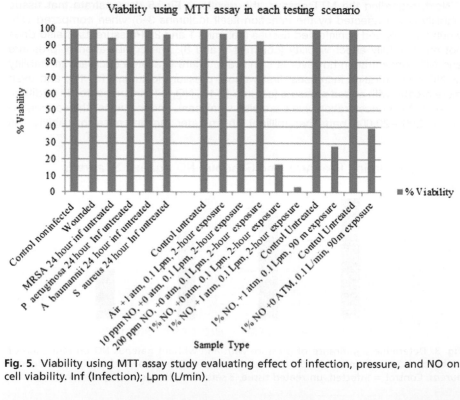

Fig. 5. Viability using MTT assay study evaluating effect of infection, pressure, and NO on cell viability. Inf (Infection); Lpm (L/min).

are able to carry out without difficulties nor can they regulate their pH within a normal level. Compared with bacteria, host cells have a highly evolved nitrosative thiol detoxification pathway, which may be hampered in a closed in vitro experimental system.

With this set of information and positive data regarding the antimicrobial effect of gNOp, understanding requirements for potential human application was the next step. The feasibility of holding 14.7 psi (1 atm) of pressure onto the dermal surface around a wound seemed unlikely at best. Thus, the next set of testing would need to evaluate the antimicrobial effect of gNOp at lower pressures.

Defense advanced research projects agency study follow-up: reduced pressures

The next set of tests indicated that lower pressures could achieve the desired antimicrobial effect. **Fig. 6** shows the bacterial log-reduction of *S aureus* against gNOp at lower pressures. In the previous testing, *S aureus* proved the most difficult of the pathogens to kill (see **Fig. 4**). Given this previous result, it was used as the benchmark for evaluating whether gNOp at a lower pressure could retain its antimicrobial effect.

With these promising results of lowering the effective pressure, attention was shifted to the time of the treatment. Although 90 minutes is similar to other wound-healing treatments, such as hyperbaric oxygen therapy, quicker treatment time, if achievable, would be more feasible for patient and medical providers. Consequently, the next phase of testing was to look into an experimental design in which the shortest length of time, with the least amount of pressure added, could achieve the same results for bacteria kill.

Increased nitric oxide concentration testing

In this third set of in vitro testing, the concentration of gaseous NO was increased to 2% (20,000 ppm). With the same testing approach, gNOp with the higher NO concentration showed a powerful bactericidal effect. **Fig. 7** shows the bacterial log-reduction of the 4 multidrug-resistant bacteria tested. An important additional note is that there was complete eradication of bacteria in at least 1 sample of each pathogen. The minimum log-reduction across all bacteria strains was 3-log reduction, whereas most samples showed complete eradication of bacteria. Results specifically indicated a

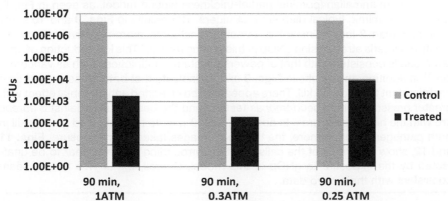

Fig. 6. Reduction of pressure and effects on bioburden. 24-hour infection, 90 minutes, 0.1 L/min flow. Control = untreated tissues, 3 sets of triplicates per experiment. Pathogen: *S aureus*.

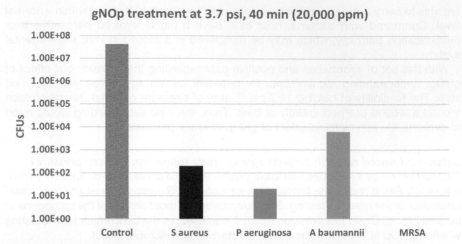

Fig. 7. Increased concentration of gaseous NO and effects on bioburden. 24-hour infection, 3.7 psi, 40 minutes, 0.1 L/min flow. Control = untreated tissues, 3 sets of triplicates per experiment. Pathogens: S aureus, P aeruginosa, A baumannii, MRSA.

10^5 to 10^7 $\log_{10}$ CFU/g reduction for strains of S aureus, P aeruginosa, with MRSA completely eradicated, whereas A baumannii achieved a 10^4 CFU/g reduction.

The results indicate gNOp, at the higher concentration, was successful in eradicating multidrug-resistant organisms. **Fig. 7** shows the effectiveness of the gNOp treatment greatly decreases bacteria load in as little as 40 minutes. **Fig. 7** also shows that even in certain bacterial strains, a 40-minute treatment is still capable of a minimum of a 3-log reduction in bioburden or greater. Both gram-negative and gram-positive bacteria appear to be susceptible to eradication using gNOp with the increase in gas concentration. One limitation is that these studies did not test anaerobes, but others have reported that gaseous NO has a similar antimicrobial effect on anaerobic bacteria.[30] These tests suggest that gNOp could be an innovative antimicrobial. The next step was to evaluate gNOp in an in vivo mammalian model to mimic typical wounds.

In Vivo Testing

Mammalian (porcine) model
The in vivo mammalian (porcine) partial-thickness wound model, as seen in **Fig. 8**, was used to mimic typical diabetic foot ulcers. The results in **Figs. 9** and **10** show a greater than 2-log antimicrobial effect against both gram-negative and gram-positive bacteria strains using gNOp in this testing model.[a] This log-reduction of bacterial load is consistent with that of powerful systemic antibiotics, such as vancomycin.[31] In addition, the results in **Figs. 9** and **10** indicate that both pressure and time are important for bacterial kill. There appears to be an added antimicrobial effect with greater pressure in the Pseudomonas testing, and the best results against S aureus are with the higher pressures. In addition, the 50-minute tests showed greater kill in both pathogens. Furthermore, the histology images taken after exposure, **Figs. 11** and **12**, show that most of the cells and the surrounding tissue appear to be unaffected by the exposure to gNOp in this model. Overall, the in vivo results seem consistent with the in vitro data.

---

[a] During the testing, the test animal expired. Standard postmortem laboratory work was conducted, including measurements for methemoglobin and known toxicology for exposure to NO. All laboratory data were within normal limits, and necropsy failed to identify the cause of death.

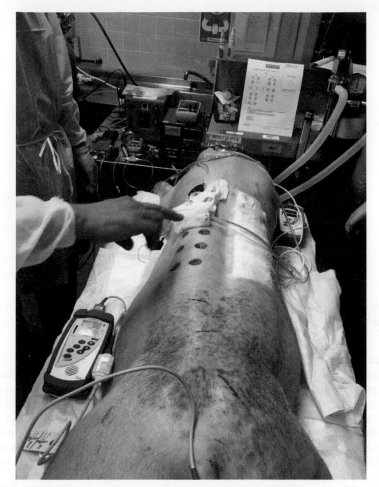

Fig. 8. Full gNOp setup in porcine mammalian partial-thickness wound model.

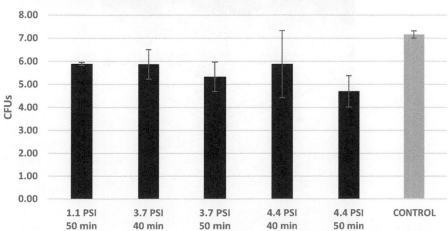

Fig. 9. In vivo mammalian model (porcine); gNOp treatment (20,000 ppm), varying pressures and times, 0.1 L/min flow; Control = untreated wounds; Pathogen: *S aureus*.

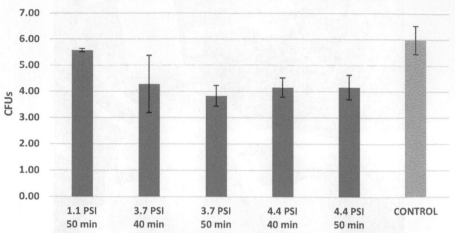

Fig. 10. In vivo mammalian model (porcine); gNOp treatment (20,000 ppm), varying pressures and times, 0.1 L/min flow; Control = untreated wounds; Pathogen: *P aeruginosa*.

Results summary

The initial DARPA proof-of-concept in vitro testing showed that gaseous NO (10,000 ppm) with added pressure (14.7 psi; 1.0 atm) was more effective killing bacteria than gaseous NO delivered without added pressure or air with pressure over a 90-minute treatment. Constant flow of gaseous NO was also essential for the bactericidal effect (0.1 L/min). With these parameters, the follow-up in vitro testing looked to achieve the same results at lower pressures. The bactericidal effect was seen at 3.7 psi (0.25 atm) and 4.4 psi (0.3 atm) over the 90-minute treatment time with the same flow and gaseous NO concentration as the initial DARPA testing. In the

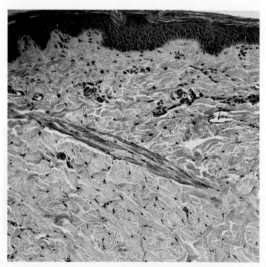

Fig. 11. Stain of pig skin that has not been exposed to gNOp (hematoxylin-eosin, original magnification ×200).

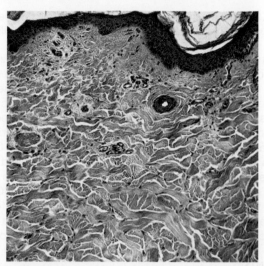

Fig. 12. Stain of pig skin that has been exposed to gNOp (hematoxylin-eosin, original magnification ×200).

increased concentration in vitro testing, gaseous NO at 20,000 ppm was administered with the goal of reducing the treatment time. Bactericidal effects were seen in the testing across pathogens at 3.7 psi (.25 atm) and a 40-minute treatment period. Finally, the parameters used in the increased concentration in vitro testing were applied in the in vivo mammalian (porcine) model. The bactericidal effect (~2-log bacterial reduction) was seen in both the gram-positive and the gram-negative pathogens.

SUMMARY

The in vitro and in vivo results show the development of gaseous NO under pressure from initial idea conception through an in vivo mammalian model. The data suggest gNOp has a powerful antimicrobial effect with potential for application in chronic and acute infections, specifically diabetic foot ulcers, or other mild to moderate skin and skin structure infections. Given the concern over antibiotic resistance, gNOp may provide an alternative solution for skin and skin structure infections over the use of standard systemic antibiotics. Traditional use of systemic antibiotics that are not organism or site specific can cause deleterious effects, propagate resistance, and require extended periods of treatment. NO presents a unique combination of properties that enable an antimicrobial effect, while reducing the likelihood of resistance issues, in a topical, localized treatment. With added pressure, gNOp enhances the bactericidal effect, especially subcutaneously where many topical treatments fail to penetrate tissues.

The histologic results in the in vitro models showed a significant viability issue with the addition of gaseous NO and the added pressure. In the in vitro model, the tissue had no way of breaking down the gaseous NO by-products (nitrites and nitrates) that cells in a living system are able to carry out without difficulties nor can they regulate their pH within a normal level. The histology images taken after exposure in the in vivo mammalian model show that most of the cells and the surrounding tissue appear to be unaffected by the exposure to gNOp. Thus, these data suggest that tissue viability in potential human models is of less concern now, after the in vivo testing, than post the in vitro testing where viability seemed to be an issue.

Looking to the future development of gNOp, additional testing will be done to optimize parameters for the best therapeutic effect and to evaluate the safety of gNOp in order to progress into potential human trials. It may also be beneficial to evaluate gNOp effect on anaerobic bacterial species. An innovative topical approach to chronic and acute wounds, like DFUs, or other skin and skin structure infections would add value to the array of existing treatment options. Avoiding the prescription of systemic antibiotics that may be of little value to certain patients, such as those with severe vascular issues, is important. A topical solution that could be used in substitution of antibiotics for these types of wounds or infections would give the medical provider an additional tool in their infection treatment tool kit. Gaseous NO under pressure has the potential to be a novel topical antimicrobial treatment for infections and may even have the ability to prevent critical colonization of bacteria before the development of an infection for any patient presenting with a chronic wound.

ACKNOWLEDGMENTS

This work was supported by DARPA grant HR0011-11-1-006, *Identify parameters for optimal delivery of pressurized nitric oxide to reduce bioburden in wound infections*; School of Podiatric Medicine's Brand Research Center and the College of Nursing and Health Sciences, Barry University, Miami Shores, Florida; Arizona School of Podiatric Medicine at Midwestern University, Glendale, Arizona; Bridge PTS, Inc, San Antonio, Texas, and REV.1 Engineering, Murrieta, California.

DISCLOSURE

The authors have a significant interest in Hansen Pharmaceutical, LLC, of which J. Jensen, J. Hanft, and S. Jensen are material owners. Hansen Pharmaceutical, LLC has paid C. Miller for consulting work. The development of gaseous NO under pressure was initially funded by a DARPA grant at Barry University, where J. Jensen, C. Miller, D. Packert, and G. Packert began work to determine the antimicrobial effects of NO. Hansen Pharmaceutical, LLC bought the intellectual property from Barry University and has continued the development of gaseous NO under pressure, which includes a significant portion of the data and information in this article. Hansen is funded through private means.

REFERENCES

1. Snyder RJ, Jensen J, Applewhite AJ, et al. A standardized approach to evaluating lower extremity chronic wounds using a checklist. Wounds 2019;31(5): S29–44. Available at: https://www.ncbi.nlm.nih.gov/pubmed/31033453.
2. Singh N, Armstrong DG, Lipsky BA. Preventing foot ulcers in patients with diabetes. JAMA 2005;293(2):217–28.
3. Margolis DJ, Kantor J, Berlin JA. Healing of diabetic neuropathic foot ulcers receiving standard treatment: a meta-analysis. Diabetes Care 1999;22(5):692–5.
4. Lavery LA, Armstrong DG, Wunderlich RP, et al. Risk factors for foot infections in individuals with diabetes. Diabetes Care 2006;29(6):1288–93.
5. Geiss LS, Li Y, Hora I, et al. Resurgence of diabetes-related nontraumatic lower-extremity amputation in the young and middle-aged adult U.S. population. Diabetes Care 2019;42(1):50–4.

6. Margolis DJ, Malay DS, Hoffstad OJ, et al. Incidence of diabetic foot ulcer and lower extremity amputation among medicare beneficiaries, 2006 to 2008. Data points #2. Rockville (MD): Agency for Healthcare Research and Quality; 2011. Data Points Publication Series [Internet]. Available at: https://www.ncbi.nlm.nih.gov/books/NBK65149/.

7. WHO, IDF. One lower limb lost to diabetes every 30 seconds, UN agency says. UN News 2005. Available at: https://news.un.org/en/story/2005/11/159922-one-lower-limb-lost-diabetes-every-30-seconds-un-agency-says.

8. IDF IDF. IDF diabetes atlas. 8th edition. Brussels (Belgium): 2017. Available at: http://www.diabetesatlas.org/. Accessed September 30, 2019.

9. Reiber GE. Epidemiology and health care costs of diabetic foot problems. In: Veves A, Giurini JM, Logerfo FW, editors. The diabetic foot. Totowa (NJ): Humana Press; 2002. p. 35–58.

10. Nussbaum SR, Carter MJ, Fife CE, et al. An economic evaluation of the impact, cost, and Medicare policy implications of chronic nonhealing wounds. Value Health 2018;21(1):27–32.

11. Barshes NR, Sigireddi M, Wrobel JS, et al. The system of care for the diabetic foot: objectives, outcomes, and opportunities. Diabet Foot Ankle 2013;4:1–12.

12. Rice JB, Desai U. Burden of diabetic foot ulcers for medicare and private insurers. Diabetes Care 2014;37(3):651–8.

13. MacKenzie EJ, Castillo RC, Jones AS, et al. Health-care costs associated with amputation or reconstruction of a limb-threatening injury. J Bone Joint Surg Am 2007;89(8):1685–92. Available at: https://journals.lww.com/jbjsjournal/Abstract/2007/08000/Health_Care_Costs_Associated_with_Amputation_or.3.aspx.

14. Raghav A, Khan ZA, Labala RK, et al. Financial burden of diabetic foot ulcers to world: a progressive topic to discuss always. Ther Adv Endocrinol Metab 2018; 9(1):29–31.

15. Pecoraro RE, Reiber GE, Burgess E. Pathways to diabetic limb amputation. Basis for prevention. Diabetes Care 1990;13(5):513–21. Available at: https://www.ncbi.nlm.nih.gov/pubmed/2351029.

16. Pecoraro RE, Ahroni JH, Boyko EJ, et al. Chronology and determinants of tissue repair in diabetic lower-extremity ulcers. Diabetes 1991;40(10):1305–13. Available at: https://www.ncbi.nlm.nih.gov/pubmed/1936593.

17. Thorpe KE, Joski P, Johnston KJ. Antibiotic-resistant infection treatment costs have doubled since 2002, now exceeding $2 billion annually. Health Aff 2018; 37(4):662–9. Available at: https://www.healthaffairs.org/doi/abs/10.1377/hlthaff.2017.1153.

18. CDC. National summary data. 2013. Available at: https://www.cdc.gov/drugresistance/pdf/3-2013-508.pdf. Accessed September 30, 2019.

19. CDC. Antibiotic Resistance Threats in the United States, 2019. Atlanta (GA): U.S. Department of Health and Human Services, CDC; 2019.

20. Jneid J, Lavigne JP, La Scola B, et al. The diabetic foot microbiota: a review. Human Microbiome Journal 2017. https://doi.org/10.1016/j.humic.2017.09.002.

21. Miller C, McMullin B, Ghaffari A, et al. Gaseous nitric oxide bactericidal activity retained during intermittent high-dose short duration exposure. Nitric Oxide 2009;20(1):16–23. Available at: https://www.sciencedirect.com/science/article/pii/S1089860308003613?via%3Dihub.

22. Ghaffari A, Jalili R, Ghaffari M, et al. Efficacy of gaseous nitric oxide in the treatment of skin and soft tissue infections. Wound Repair Regen 2007;15(3):368–77. Available at: https://onlinelibrary.wiley.com/doi/abs/10.1111/j.1524-475X.2007.00239.x.

23. Privett BJ, Broadnax AD, Bauman SJ, et al. Examination of bacterial resistance to exogenous nitric oxide. Nitric Oxide 2012;26(3):169–73.
24. Barraud N, Hassett DJ, Hwang S, et al. Involvement of nitric oxide in biofilm dispersal of pseudomonas aeruginosa. J Bacteriol 2006;188(21):7344–53.
25. Rezakhanlou AM, Miller C, McMullin B, et al. Gaseous nitric oxide exhibits minimal effect on skin fibroblast extracellular matrix gene expression and immune cell viability. Cell Biol Int 2011;35(4):407–15. Available at: https://onlinelibrary.wiley.com/doi/abs/10.1042/CBI20100420.
26. Witte MB, Kiyama T, Barbul A. Nitric oxide enhances experimental wound healing in diabetes. Br J Surg 2002;89(12):1594–601. Available at: https://www.ncbi.nlm.nih.gov/pubmed/12445072.
27. Jones ML, Ganopolsky JG, Labbe A, et al. Antimicrobial properties of nitric oxide and its application in antimicrobial formulations and medical devices. Appl Microbiol Biotechnol 2010;88(2):401–7. Available at: https://www.ncbi.nlm.nih.gov/pubmed/20680266.
28. Ghaffari A, Neil DH, Ardakani A, et al. A direct nitric oxide gas delivery system for bacterial and mammalian cell cultures. Nitric Oxide 2005;12(3):129–40. Available at: https://www.ncbi.nlm.nih.gov/pubmed/15797841.
29. Miller C, Miller MK, Ghaffari A, et al. Treatment of chronic nonhealing leg ulceration with gaseous nitric oxide: a case study. J Cutan Med Surg 2004;8(4):233–8. Available at: https://www.ncbi.nlm.nih.gov/pubmed/16092001.
30. Reighard KP, Schoenfisch MH. Antibacterial action of nitric oxide-releasing chitosan oligosaccharides against Pseudomonas aeruginosa under aerobic and anaerobic conditions. Antimicrobial Agents Chemother 2015;59(10):6506–13.
31. Moise PA, Sakoulas G, Forrest A, et al. Vancomycin in vitro bactericidal activity and its relationship to efficacy in clearance of methicillin-resistant Staphylococcus aureus bacteremia. Antimicrobial Agents Chemother 2007;51(7):2582–6.

III. Temple University School of Podiatric Medicine

III. Temple Univeristy School of
Podiatric Medicine

Charcot Reconstruction
Understanding and Treating the Deformed Charcot Neuropathic Arthropathic Foot

Kwasi Y. Kwaadu, DPM

KEYWORDS

- Amputation • Charcot neuroarthropathy • Charcot neuropathic arthropathy
- Diabetes • Diabetic foot deformity • Equinus • Superconstructs

KEY POINTS

- Confirm perfusion prior to reconstruction.
- Isolate and dorsiflex the hindfoot exclusively during the equinal correction.
- Include the subtalar joint with the talonavicular joint arthrodesis.
- Incorporate a blocking screw in the medial column plate, just distal to the head of the medial column bolt.
- Reconstruction does not obviate future surgery or bracing.

 Video content accompanies this article at http://www.podiatric.theclinics.com.

INTRODUCTION

Originally described by William Musgrave in 1703 and further elaborated on by Jean-Martin Charcot in 1868, Charcot neuropathic arthropathy (CNA) is a neuropathically mediated destruction of the bones and joints of the foot that can lead to a rocker-bottom collapsed deformity primarily clustered about the tarsometatarsal and naviculocuneiform joints.[1,2] When the deformity extends proximally to involve the tibiotalocalcaneal articulations, the deformity becomes even more difficult to manage conservatively.[1] These destructive changes can lead to ulceration and potentially amputation. Despite its long history, a clear and definitive understanding of the disease etiology is still lacking. Charcot described the neuropathy and associated it with degeneration of the central nervous system from damage to "trophic centers" in anterior horn cells, leading to a neurogenic deficit in bone nutrition and ultimately ataxic neuropathically mediated vascular dysregulation.[1] And in the twentieth century, his

Department of Surgery, Temple University School of Podiatric Medicine, 148 North 8th Street, Philadelphia, PA 19107, USA
E-mail address: kkwaadu@gmail.com

Clin Podiatr Med Surg 37 (2020) 247–261
https://doi.org/10.1016/j.cpm.2019.12.002
0891-8422/20/© 2019 Elsevier Inc. All rights reserved.
podiatric.theclinics.com

hypothesis was replaced with 2 current working theories: the neurotraumatic and neurovascular theories.[3–5]

The 2 current theories assert that microtrauma to the insensate foot combined with increase vascular perfusion, as a secondary consequence of neurologically mediated sympathectomy, results in a loss of autonomic innervation to arterial perfusion. In 1936, William Riley Jordan described CNA as a complication of diabetic neuropathy and was the first to formally publish the association. The overall incidence of CNA in the general diabetic population has been reported less than 1%, but is upward of 13% in those with neuropathy.[6] Compared with the general population, diabetics with neuropathy are overwhelmingly afflicted; however, any patient with neuropathy could be at risk. And although neuropathy and diabetes as major risk factors, a clear definitive understanding of the etiology of the disease is still lacking.

PATHOGENESIS

The current pathogenesis of the etiology has shifted more toward an osteoclast-osteoblast imbalance. In the presence or absence of associated radiographic osteolysis, an erythematous and edematous foot with temperature difference greater than 2°C compared with the contralateral site with associated local inflammation defines the acute phase clinically (**Fig. 1**). The associated inflammation has historically been viewed as a result of the disease process, largely as a secondary consequence of unchecked and uninterrupted microtrauma to the insensate limb. Jeffcoate[7] hypothesized, however, that an exaggerated inflammatory response to trauma, obvious or otherwise, could trigger an inflammatory cascaded through the increased expression of proinflammatory cytokines, with particular emphasis on interleukin (IL)-1, resulting in increased osteoclastic activity. This activation then leads to osteolysis, fracture, further potentiating the inflammatory process via the receptor activator of nuclear factor kappa-β ligand (RANK-L) pathway. This RANK-L pathway has been demonstrated active in other lytic-mediated disease states, such as osteoporosis, inflammatory arthridities, malignancy, and Paget disease.[8] Uccioli and colleagues[9] utilized a novel fluorescence-activated cell sorter analysis and were able to demonstrate an increase in an inflammatory phenotype of circulating monocytes exhibiting an increase in the production of proinflammatory cytokines, such as tumor necrosis factor alpha α, interleukin (IL)-1β, and IL-6, in patients with CNA, compared with diabetic controls and healthy subjects without CNA. Furthermore, these values were demonstrated to decrease after fracture resolution and convalescence. Mabilleau and colleagues[10] investigated the influence of RANK-L on monocytes in 9 diabetic Charcot patients. Although there was a baseline increase in osteoclastic activity in Charcot patients compared with diabetic and healthy controls, there was an appreciably significant increase in osteoclastic activity with the addition of the RANK-L.

The process reveals an association with an increase in the systemic levels of inflammatory biomarkers associated with osseous metabolism, further demonstrating that inflammation may not merely be a symptom of the disease, but potentially the cause.

Denosumab (Prolia, Amgen, California), a RANK-L antibody used in the treatment of osteoporosis, has been studied, demonstrating CNA fracture resolution over a shorter duration compared with controls, further entrenching current suspicion about the influence of the RANK-L pathway.[11]

This collective of research continues to move in the direction of formally unmasking the physiologic cause(s) of CNA, with the hope of preemptively modulating and ultimately preventing the unabated osteolysis that can lead to catastrophic collapse with residual deformity at risk for ulceration and amputation.

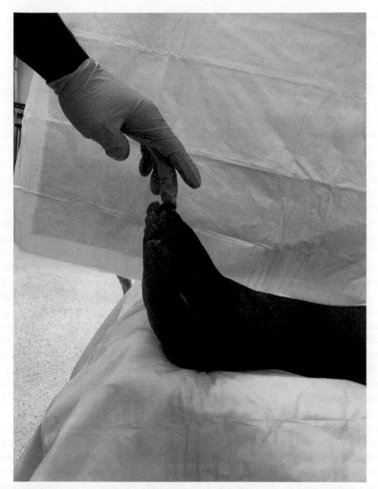

Fig. 1. A clinical appearance of the edematous and deformed acute CNA foot.

Bisphosphonates also have been studied in an attempt to halt the unabated osteolysis. These antiresorptive medications have demonstrated efficacy in osteoporosis and other osteoclastic-mediated disease states. Although they have been demonstrated to decrease inflammatory markers and decrease bone turnover. In the setting of acute CNA, however, there is little evidence demonstrating clear benefit in resolution of the pathogenesis with respect to the endpoint of mitigation of the destruction and the preservation of function.[8,12,13]

Bone stimulators, ultrasonographic and electric, are adjunctive therapies used to assist in delayed bone healing. And although intuitively reasonable, there is little evidence to formally support its utility and efficacy in mitigating the osteolysis associated with acute CNA. When used, they primarily serve as adjunctive therapy to postsurgical reconstruction.[14–16] Moreover, their renal implications should caution indiscriminate use.

SURGICAL MANAGEMENT

Although a large majority of patients with CNA undergo these destructive articular changes as a secondary consequence of diabetic neuropathy, not all patients with

CNA are diabetic. And because of this generally low prevalence, there are no studies comparing outcomes between the 2 patient groups. Nevertheless, the associated sequelae of diabetes and its implication on cellular and organ function add an increased layer of complication that ultimately could confound outcomes.[3,4,6] Thus, in the diabetic population, patient intake requires comprehensive investigation in order to ascertain whether surgical reconstruction is in the patient's interests, juxtaposed with any preexisting comorbidities.[3,4]

There is a historic misconception that perfusion in CNA is largely unaffected. Historically published reports consistently noted this aspect of perfusion as so generous, it has been described as bounding, as a sequela of the neurologically mediated sympathectomy, resulting in a loss of autonomic innervation to arterial perfusion.[1–6] Because diabetes also is associated with peripheral and cardiovascular disease, however, confirmation of perfusion is a critical aspect of the patient work-up in preparation for reconstruction and must not be overestimated.[17–20]

It is important to recognized that although surgical reconstruction may correlate with a comparably improved quality of life, not all patients are served well with surgery.[19,20] Rettedal and colleagues[21] used prognostic scoring systems used to aid in the surgical decision making, correlating a lower score with a decreased ulcer recurrence and amputation after reconstruction. The score and risk factors were demonstrated to increase with age, body mass index, presence of wound or osteomyelitis, location of involvement, activity of the disease, and elevated hemoglobin A_{1c}.

Increases in the level of glycosylated hemoglobin above 8 mg/dL have been associated with increased risk of operative complications.[22] Although important, the risks of treatment should be juxtaposed to the risks of not treating. A patient with a deformity with an ulceration at risk for infection or impending ulceration should not be declined reconstruction exclusively because of an elevated glycosylated hemoglobin level. The possibility of deep infection and amputation as a consequence of delayed reconstruction may outweigh the concern for perioperative complication.

The indication for reconstruction surgery generally include an unbraceable limb-threatening deformity, unstable joints with tenting of the surrounding soft tissues, and recalcitrant ulceration in the presence or absence osteomyelitis (**Fig. 2**). Although agreement exist with respect to the general goals, the techniques are not standardized and frankly are difficult to standardize. This difficulty influenced by the different architectural endpoints of the deformity prior to reconstruction. And, because the pathology and associated deformity can occur at different articular segments in the midfoot and hindfoot, unlike with hallux valgus reconstruction, where the preoperative magnitude of deformity may provide some guidance into the procedure of choice, there are no specific or standardized approaches definitively correlating levels of reconstruction with respect to the magnitude of the preoperative deformity. Consequently, this somewhat subjective component to the management of an already profoundly complex musculoskeletal pathology adds variability to an already elusive endpoint. Nonetheless, without intervention, the natural course is progressive articula and osseous destruction, further exacerbating deformity and increasing risk of ulceration, infection, and amputation, endpoints that have a direct impact on quality of life.[4] Thus, the intent of reconstruction is to intervene prior to failure of the surrounding soft tissues, increasing risk for amputation, in order to help mitigate the associated cardiovascular risks and mortality associated with the new increase in work demand.

The Elchenholtz classification, a 3-stage classification system describing the radiographic progression of the deformity from acute fragmentation and dislocation to coalescence, and finally to maturation and remodeling to sclerotic bone, has been used to largely communicate the deformity type with respect to timing of surgical

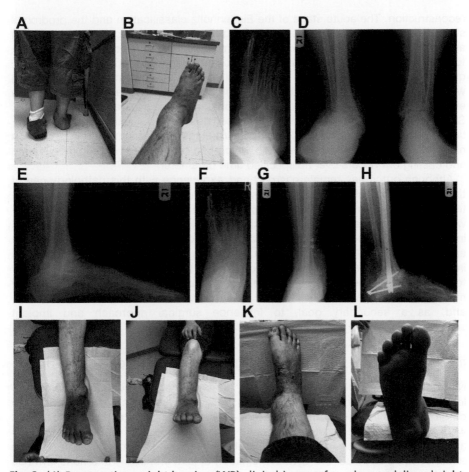

Fig. 2. (*A*) Preoperative weight-bearing (WB) clinical image of a valgus malaligned right ankle and hindfoot. (*B*) Preoperative non-WB clinical image of a valgus malaligned right ankle and hindfoot. (*C*) Preoperative WB dorsoplantar (DP) radiograph of the valgus malaligned right ankle and hindfoot. (*D*) Preoperative WB bilateral ankle anteroposterior (AP) radiograph demonstrating a valgus malaligned right ankle with retained hardware and a rectus-aligned left ankle. (*E*) Preoperative WB lateral radiograph of the valgus malaligned right ankle with retained hardware. (*F*) Postoperative WB DP radiograph of the reconstructed and realigned previously malaligned valgus right ankle and hindfoot. (*G*) Postoperative WB AP ankle/tibia radiograph of the reconstructed and realigned previously malaligned valgus right ankle and hindfoot with intramedullary fixation. (*H*) Postoperative WB lateral ankle/tibia radiograph of the reconstructed and realigned previously malaligned valgus right ankle and hindfoot with intramedullary fixation. (*I*) Postoperative AP clinical image of the reconstructed and realigned previously malaligned valgus right ankle and hindfoot with intramedullary fixation. (*J*) Modified postoperative AP clinical image of the reconstructed and realigned previously malaligned valgus right ankle and hindfoot with intramedullary fixation. (*K*) Modified postoperative AP clinical image, taken from the cranial to caudal direction, of the reconstructed and realigned previously malaligned valgus right ankle and hindfoot with intramedullary fixation. (*L*) Postoperative clinical image of the plantar foot of the reconstructed and realigned previously malaligned valgus right ankle and hindfoot with intramedullary fixation.

reconstruction. The acute stage of the Eichenholtz classification and the prodromal stage 0, later added by Shibata and colleagues, emphasizing clinical inflammation and edema even in the absence of radiographic fragmentation and collapse, have historically been regarded as the time to avoid formal open reduction largely as a consequence of osteopenia reducing hardware purchase and inflammation complicating wound healing.[2,6] And although there are studies describing successful reconstruction even in the acute phase, formal reconstruction generally is avoided during this stage. Staged reconstruction in these cases have been described but, ultimately, reconstruction is preferentially performed during the third stage when edema and inflammation have fully resolved, the duration within which can be mitigated with immobilization and casting but occurs over no specified time parameter.[5,6,23–25]

Although outcomes remain guarded and experience with this pathology can at times appear outright unpredictable, there is evidence that successful reconstruction can improve patient quality of life by reducing ulcer risk and may improve footwear choices. And although more proximal pathology is associated with increased instability, there is no clear evidence that Charcot deformities at particular locations are associated with improved or worse prognoses after reconstruction (**Fig. 3**). The implication of the location of the pathology largely focuses on identification, in order to increase the awareness of the pathology, because Charcot has been historically misdiagnosed, largely due to the relatively low prevalence in the general population, and, as a secondary goal, to influence surgical approach and implant selection[1,6,8,26]

RECONSTRUCTION OF CHARCOT NEUROPATHIC ARTHROPATHY OF THE MIDFOOT

Neuropathic arthropathic collapse primarily affecting the tarsometatarsal and naviculocuneiform joints, a finding corroborated in most of the anatomic classifications of the deformity, is influenced by the cantilever bending forces in the midfoot exacerbated with continued weight bearing. This results in plantarflexion of the anterior calcaneus and the midfoot, increasing plantar midfoot pressures and ulcer risk.[3–6] The additive effect of equinus, influenced by a combination of joint immobility and nonenzymatic glycation of the tendons and surrounding soft tissues, further exacerbates the pathology.[27,28] Consequently, a critical aspect of the reconstruction of Charcot with midfoot collapse is relieving this deforming force of the achilles tendon by lengthening via the Hoke triple hemisection procedure.[5] Thereafter, a percutaneous 5-mm Schanz pin placed in the calcaneus, from posterior to anterior, can be used to facilitate formal lengthening of the tendon by plantarflexing the posterior arm of the Schanz pin. The use of the Schanz pin is crucial. The traditional maneuver of dorsiflexing the foot to facilitate lengthening does not work effectively secondary to the midfoot collapse and uncoupling associated with this deformity (**Fig. 4**). Consequently, dorsiflexing the foot in this scenario results in undercorrection of the hindfoot equinus. A gastrocnemius recession is an underpowered procedure with these deformities and can result in undercorrection and an increased risk of recurrence of the hindfoot equinus.[27–29] Following this maneuver, percutaneously inserted Steinmann pins are used to provisionally transfixate the ankle joint to maintain the correction. With the equinus corrected, the Schanz pin is removed and attention then is directed to the midfoot, where deformity correction can proceed, building the complex puzzle to the new rectus aligned hindfoot. A medial utility incision allows access of all the medial column joints, facilitating articular preparation and deformity correction, along with plate fixation as needed. A traditional lateral triple arthrodesis incision allows access to the subtalar joint, the calcaneocuboid joint, and the lateral fourth and fifth tarsometatarsal

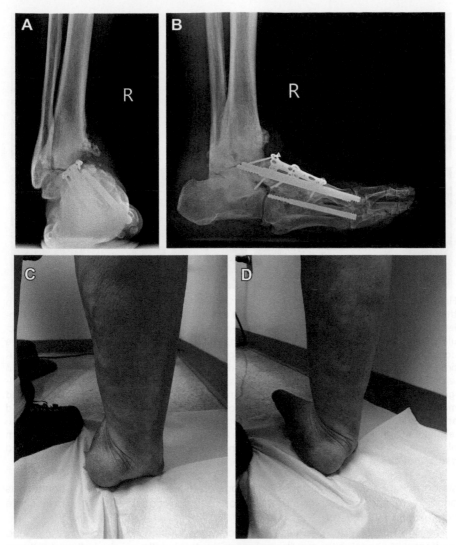

Fig. 3. (*A*) Anteroposterior ankle radiograph of a prior midfoot CNA reconstruction with new CNA at the ankle with varus malalignment. (*B*) Lateral ankle radiograph of a prior mid-foot CNA reconstruction with new CNA at the ankle with varus malalignment. (*C*) Clinical weight-bearing (WB) image of the ankle taken from directly posterior with varus malalignment. (*D*) Clinical WB image of the ankle taken from a posteromedial direction with varus malalignment of the hindfoot.

joints to facilitate articular preparation. These incisions also can facilitate through and through corrective osteotomies in cases of largely coalesced deformity without clear and discrete anatomic joints.

Formal articular preparation may reduce nonunion risk. Hand instrumentation, such as curettes and curved osteotomes, are ideal for articular take downs to the underlying subchondral plate because they generate less heat that power instrumentation (**Fig. 5**). Nonetheless, power instrumentation is safely used with irrigation to reduce heat generation Thereafter, fenestration the underlying

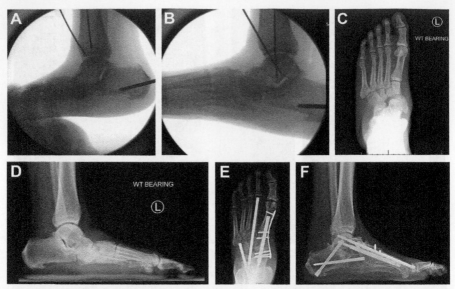

Fig. 4. (*A*) Lateral fluoroscopic projection of the ankle in equinus, with temporary pins in the tibia and the correcting lever (Schanz pin) in the calcaneus. (*B*) Lateral fluoroscopic projection of the corrected ankle equinus, with temporary pins transfixating the tibiotalar articulation, and the correcting lever (Schanz pin) still within the calcaneus. (*C*) Preoperative dorsoplantar radiograph demonstrating naviculocuneiform dislocation as part of the CNA process. (*D*) Preoperative lateral radiograph demonstrating naviculocuneiform dislocation with plantarflexion as part of the CNA process. (*E*) Postoperative DP radiograph of the realigned and reconstructed malalignment with intramedullary fixation in the first and second metatarsals, a medial column plate, and a noncannulated bolt across the calcaneocuboid arthrodesis site. (*F*) Postoperative lateral radiograph of the realigned and reconstructed malalignment with intramedullary fixation in the first and second metatarsals, a medial column plate, a noncannulated bolt across the calcaneocuboid arthrodesis site, and a cannulated partially threaded screw across the subtalar arthrodesis site.

subchondral plate has the benefit of exposing more of the underlying cancellous bone, increasing osseous perfusion across the arthrodesis site to help facilitate consolidation (Video 1).

The talonavicular arthrodesis site is reduced by pronating the forefoot on the pinned hindfoot and engaging the windlass mechanism by dorsiflexing the hallux in order to try to recreate the medial longitudinal arch if possible (if the deformity has spared the overall architecture of the talonavicular joint) (Video 2). After reduction, the talonavicular joint and the posterior subtalar joints are provisionally pinned, in preparation for fixation. Even when the midfoot CNA does not formerly involve the posterior subtalar joint, including subtalar joint arthrodesis helps increase the consolidated osseous hindfoot bulk and recruit calcaneal perfusion, in order to avoid concentrating hardware in the talus, potentially compromising talar perfusion and viability.[30]

Current guidelines in reconstruction recommend (1) extending the arthrodesis far beyond the zone of injury in order to maximize contact between the fixation and good bone not compromised by the disease, (2) resection of underlying bone in order to shorten the underlying osseous architecture to facilitate reconstruction without increase soft tissue tension, (3) the utilization of the strongest fixation device without further compromising soft tissues, and (4) fixation devices placed in biomechanically optimal locations.[31–36] Intramedullary bolts are excellent fixation choices

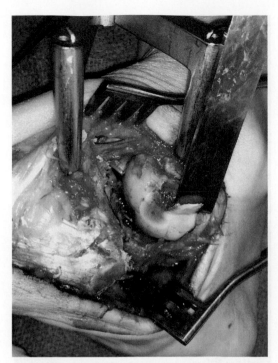

Fig. 5. Hand resection of joints in preparation for formal arthrodesis.

that can be delivered through small incision, limiting the additional soft tissue dissection and exposure. These intramedullary devices are mechanically optimal because they resist cantilever bending forces that could gap the plantar aspects of the reconstruction, increasing risk of dorsal malunion and valgus deformity recurrence.[34–36] These intramedullary bolts can be delivered in retrograde fashion from the metatarsophalangeal joints into the talus. As part of the preoperative work-up, the width of the metatarsal canal should be confirmed preoperatively on digital radiography, if possible, to confirm accommodation for the width of the corresponding bolt. Current intramedullary bolts options are 6.5 mm, used more commonly in the first metatarsal, and the 5.0 mm in diameter bolt, more commonly used in the lesser metatarsal. The medial column fixation can be supplemented with a medial locking plate. A blocking screw can be used in the distal aspect of this plate to further limit micromotion along the medial column that potentially could result in motion of the medial column bolt and increase risk of hardware failure and/or nonunion. In order to accomplish this, the measured length of the beam is shortened by 2 mm to 3 cm in order that there remains real estate to accommodate this blocking screw, to avoid crowding with the head of the intramedullary beam. Consequently, and in preparation for placement of this blocking screw, the medial column bolt is advanced, when initially inserted, further beyond the level of the metatarsal head, to ultimately terminate at the midshaft level of the first metatarsal (**Fig. 6**). Although these plates increase mechanical stability, they increase the underlying bulk and might not be feasible in thin skin. Fortunately, the intraosseous position of these biomechanically optimal bolts spares hardware exposure in cases of delayed wound healing that could potentially compromise the underlying hardware.[31–36]

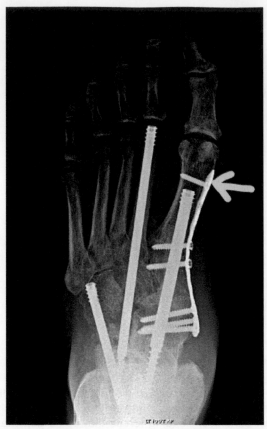

Fig. 6. Postsurgical CNA reconstruction with *blue arrow* demonstrating the blocking screw placed transversely in the most distal screw hole in the medial column plate.

When the deformity extends to the ankle and posterior subtalar joints, reconstruction can be approached with a lateral curvilinear incision with resection of the lateral malleolus (**Fig. 7**). Fixation options included intramedullary nailing and locked or blade plating, with or without external fixation. In the presence of compromised soft tissues laterally, a prone posterior approach can be used. Through the posterior approach, the Achilles is transected on entry and primarily repaired with nonabsorbable suture during closure. Both approaches allow formal access to the tibiotalar and posterior subtalar joints.

Particularly in the presence of prior reconstruction but even in the absence thereof, infection must be ruled out in the presence of osteolysis of the talus/hindfoot (**Fig. 8**). Inflammatory markers, erythrocyte sedimentation rate, and C-reactive protein level along with complete blood cell counts with differential should be obtained. As the pathogenesis involves inflammation, laboratory data may at times be equivocal. In these instances, a bone biopsy and culture may provide useful information. If the collective of information trends toward infection, the infected osseous segment is resected and an antibiotic cement spacer can be placed temporarily. The patient then is treated with antibiotics targeted to the infecting organism over the course of 6 weeks to 8 weeks or per the recommendation of the infectious disease physician. The baseline high-risk nature of this disease pathology and scenario is served well

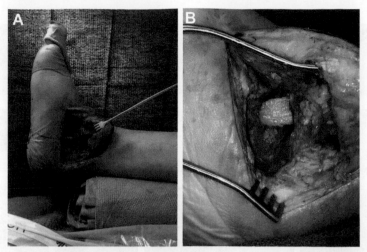

Fig. 7. (*A*) Intraoperative clinical picture demonstrating the lateral hindfoot incision used for the tibiocalcaneal arthrodesis. (*B*) Intraoperative clinical picture demonstrating the lateral hindfoot incision used for the tibiocalcaneal arthrodesis, demonstrating the interposing resected fibula autograft.

with a formal consultation. Pending infection resolution, the antibiotic spacer is removed and reconstruction can proceed (see **Fig. 8**).

Reconstruction to a predeformity architecture is not a consistently realistic endpoint and attempting this invariably adds additional time to an already time-consuming operation. The surgeon should have a low threshold for excising and remove bone that may inhibit deformity reduction, in order to reduce tension on the soft tissues.

Utilization of allogenic bone grafts is commonplace in osseous reconstruction. The utilization of large nonviable grafts in CNA reconstruction, however, warrants rethinking. Firstly, it violates Sammarco's second point of CNA reconstruction advocating the resection of underlying bone in order to shorten the underlying osseous architecture to facilitate reconstruction without increases soft tissue tension.[31] Secondly, and from a physiologic perspective, the recognition of CNA as a disease involving an osteoclastic imbalance creates a scenario where the utilization of these nonviable allogenic bone grafts could foster an environment less likely to collectively promote osseous consolidation, potentially increasing nonunion risk, hardware failure, deformity recurrence, ulceration, infection, and ultimately amputation.

An equally important aspect of CNA reconstruction is soft tissue handling and closure. Negative-pressure wound therapy (NPWT) has demonstrated significant utility in the management of chronic wounds. The accelerated healing has been described as a result of improved perfusion through the reduction of interstitial edema and increased rate of granulation tissue formation as a result of mechanical stress.[37,38] Although the NPWT system was designed for the accelerated healing of chronic wounds, the use of this device has been advocated in reducing soft tissue complications after acute skeletal trauma, demonstrating utility in compromised soft tissues, primarily in the traumatic setting. These benefits of NPWT conferred toward resuscitation of traumatized tissue are worth considering in this setting.[39–42]

After reconstruction, close monitoring is necessary. Postsurgical complications have been reported to exceed greater than 50%[1–6,8,18,23,26,43] (see **Fig. 8**). The following risk factors have been associated with major amputation after Charcot reconstruction: postoperative nonunion, development of CNA at new

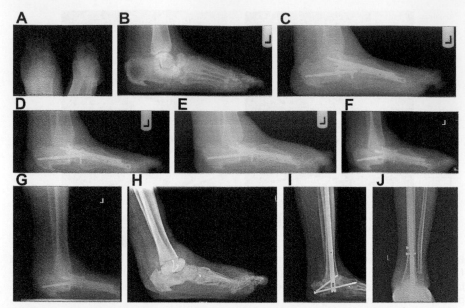

Fig. 8. (*A*) Preoperative bilateral weight-bearing (WB) dorsoplantar radiographs demonstrating superimposition of the left talonavicular articulation and the left calcaneocuboid articulation, indicative of dislocation of each of the aforementioned joints. (*B*) Preoperative WB lateral radiograph demonstrating dislocation of the talonavicular and calcaneocuboid articulations, with associated plantarflexion of the talus and calcaneus. (*C*) Postoperative WB lateral radiograph demonstrating realignment arthrodesis of the talonavicular and calcaneocuboid joints. (*D*) Lateral ankle radiograph demonstrating the initiation of talar body osteolysis. (*E*). Lateral ankle radiograph demonstrating the progression of talar body osteolysis. (*F*) Lateral ankle radiograph demonstrating further progression of talar body osteolysis. (*G*) Lateral tibia radiograph demonstrating even further progression of talar body osteolysis. (*H*) Lateral ankle radiograph demonstrating interval placement of antibiotic cement in the ankle mortise after interval resection of the osteolytic talar body. (*I*) WB lateral ankle/tibia radiograph of the tibiocalcaneal arthrodesis with intramedullary fixation with incorporation of the fibular autograft. (*J*) WB anteroposterior ankle/tibia radiograph of the tibiocalcaneal arthrodesis with intramedullary fixation.

locations, peripheral arterial disease, renal disease, delayed postoperative healing, postoperative osteomyelitis, and elevated hemoglobin A_{1c}.[1–6,8,18,20–22]

Reconstruction improves the general foot architecture but it neither reverses the destruction nor permanently obviates the use of custom molded ankle foot orthoses or other similarly custom molded bracing.[5,44,45] The analogy to facilitate patient education is that the irreversible nature of CNA is not unlike poor vision that permanently requires some vision-enhancing adjunct (glasses or contact lenses) to facilitate utility and function.

SUMMARY

Few patients, when initially diagnosed, truly comprehend how devastating a pathology this is and generally believe that surgery will simply fix their problem. The CNA deformity is a life-altering diagnosis, however, with an inherent level of unpredictability that can be psychologically overwhelming to the infirmed over the course of treatment. The surgical work-up and technical aspects of reconstruction are critical for any possibility of success. Consequently, the management of CNA and its associated complications requires a heightened level intellectual and an emotional maturity, supplemented with constant patient education.

DISCLOSURE

The author has no financial conflicts to disclose.

SUPPLEMENTARY DATA

Supplementary data related to this article can be found online at https://doi.org/10.1016/j.cpm.2019.12.002.

REFERENCES

1. Varma AK. Charcot neuroarthropathy of the foot an ankle: a review. J Foot Ankle Surg 2013;52(6):740–9.
2. Saltzman CL. Ankle arthritis. In: Coughlin MJ, Mann RA, Saltzman CL, editors. Surgery of the foot and ankle. 8th edition. Philadelphia: Mosby; 2007. p. p923–84.
3. Sohn MW, Lee TA, Stuck RM, et al. Mortality risk of Charcot arthropathy compared with that of diabetic foot ulcer and diabetes alone. Diabetes Care 2009;32(5): 816–21.
4. Pakarinen TK, Laine HJ, Maenpaa H, et al. Long-term outcome and quality of life in patients with Charcot foot. Foot Ankle Surg 2009;15(4):187–91.
5. Brodsky JW. The diabetic foot. In: Coughlin MJ, Mann RA, Saltzman CL, editors. Surgery of the foot and ankle. 8th edition. Philadelphia: Mosby; 2007. p. p1281–368.
6. Wukich DK, Sung W. Charcot arthropathy of the foot and ankle: modern concepts and management review. J Diabetes Complications 2009;23(6):409–26.
7. Jeffcoate W. The causes of the Charcot syndrome. Clin Podiatr Med Surg 2008; 25(1):29–42.
8. Botek G, Figas S, Narra S. Charcot neuroarthropathy advances. understanding pathogenesis and medical and surgical treatment. Clin Podiatr Med Surg 2019; 36(4):663–84.
9. Uccioli L, Sinistro A, Almerighi C, et al. Proinflammatory modulation of the surface and cytokine phenotype of monocytes in patients with acute Charcot foot. Diabetes Care 2010;33(2):350–5.
10. Mabilleau G, Petrova NL, Edmonds ME, et al. Increased osteoclastic activity in acute Charcot's osteoarthropathy: the role of receptor activator of nuclear factor-kappaB ligand. Diabetologia 2008;51(6):1035–40.
11. Busch-Westbroek TE, Delpeut K, Balm R, et al. Effect of single dose of RANKL antibody treatment on acute Charcot neuro-osteoarthropathy of the foot. Diabetes Care 2018;41(3):e21–2.
12. Jeffcoate WJ. Charcot foot syndrome. Diabet Med 2015;32(6):760–70.
13. Richard JL, Almasri M, Schuldiner S. Treatment of active Charcot foot with bisphosphonates: a systematic review of the literature. Diabetologia 2012;55(5): 1258–64.
14. Petrisor B, Lau JT. Electrical bone stimulation: an overview and its use in high risk and Charcot foot and ankle reconstructions. Foot Ankle Clin 2005;10(4):609–20.
15. Saxena A, DiDomenico LA, Widtfeldt A, et al. Implantable electrical bone stimulation for arthrodesis of the foot and ankle in high-risk patients: a multicenter study. J Foot Ankle Surg 2005;44(6):450–4.

16. Strauss E, Gonya G. Adjunct low intensity ultrasound in Charcot neuroarthropathy. Clin Orthop Relat Res 1998;349:132–8.
17. Wukich DK, Raspovic KM, Hobizal KB, et al. Radiographic analysis of diabetic midfoot Charcot neuroarthropathy with and without midfoot ulceration. Foot Ankle Int 2014;35(11):1108–15.
18. Chang BB, Shah DM, Darling RC III, et al. Treatment of the diabetic foot from a vascular surgeon's viewpoint. Clin Orthop Relat Res 1993;296:27–30.
19. Wukich DK, Sadoskas D, Vaudreuil NJ, et al. Comparison of diabetic Charcot patients with and without foot wounds. Foot Ankle Int 2017;38(2):140–8.
20. Elmarsafi T, Anghel EL, Sinkin J, et al. Risk factors associated with major lower extremity amputation after osseous diabetic Charcot reconstruction. J Foot Ankle Surg 2019;58(2):295–300.
21. Rettedal D, Parker A, Popchak A, et al. Prognostic scoring system for patients undergoing reconstructive foot and ankle surgery for Charcot neuroarthropathy: the Charcot reconstruction preoperative prognostic score. J Foot Ankle Surg 2018; 57(3):451–5.
22. Wukich DK, Crim BE, Frykberg RG, et al. Neuropathy and poorly controlled diabetes increase the rate of surgical site infection after foot and ankle surgery. J Bone Joint Surg Am 2014;96(10):832–9.
23. Frykberg RG, Zgonis T, Armstrong DG, et al. Diabetic foot disorders. A clinical practice guideline (2006 revision). J Foot Ankle Surg 2006;45(5 Suppl):S1–66.
24. Burns PR, Wukich DK. Surgical reconstruction of the Charcot rearfoot and ankle. Clin Podiatr Med Surg 2008;25(1):95–120.
25. Simon SR, Tejwani SG, Wilson DL, et al. Arthrodesis as an early alternative to nonoperative management of Charcot arthropathy of the diabetic foot. J Bone Joint Surg Am 2000;82-A(7):939–50.
26. Labovitz JM, Shapiro JM, Satterfield VK, et al. Excess cost and healthcare resources associated with delayed diagnosis of Charcot foot. J Foot Ankle Surg 2018;57(5):952–6.
27. Frykberg RG, Bowen J, Hall J, et al. Prevalence of equinus in diabetic versus nondiabetic patients. J Am Podiatr Med Assoc 2012;102(2):84–8.
28. Reddy GK. Cross-linking in collagen by nonenzymatic glycation increases the matrix stiffness in rabbit Achilles tendon. Exp Diabesity Res 2004;5(2):143–53.
29. Greenhagen RM, Johnson AR, Bevilacqua NJ. Gastrocnemius recession or tendo-achilles lengthening for equinus deformity in the diabetic foot? Clin Podiatr Med Surg 2012;29(3):413–24.
30. Miller AN, Prasarn ML, Dyke JP, et al. Quantitative assessment of the vascularity of the talus with gadolinium-enhanced magnetic resonance imaging. J Bone Joint Surg Am 2011;93-A(12):1116–21.
31. Sammarco VJ. Superconstructs in the treatment of Charcot foot deformity: plantar plating, locked plating, and axial screw fixation. Foot Ankle Clin 2009;14(3): 393–407.
32. Marks RM, Parks BG, Schon LC. Midfoot fusion technique for neuroarthropathic feet: biomechanical analysis and rationale. Foot Ankle Int 1998;19(8):507–10.
33. Schneekloth BJ, Lowery NJ, Wukich DK. Charcot neuroarthropathy in patients with diabetes: an updated systematic review of surgical management. J Foot Ankle Surg 2016;55(3):586–90.
34. Lamm BM, Siddiqui NA, Nair AK, et al. Intramedullary foot fixation for midfoot Charcot neuroarthropathy. J Foot Ankle Surg 2012;51(4):531–6.
35. Kann JN, Parks BG, Schon LC. Biomechanical evaluation of two different screw positions for fusion of the calcaneocuboid joint. Foot Ankle Int 1999;20(1):33–6.

36. Sammarco GJ. Diabetic arthropathy. In: Sammarco GJ, editor. The foot in diabetes. Philadelphia: Lea and Febiger; 1991. p. 153–72.

37. Argenta LC, Morykwas MJ. Vacuum-assisted closure: a new method for wound control and treatment: clinical experience. Ann Plast Surg 1997;38(6):563–76.

38. Morykwas MJ, Argenta LC, Shelton-Brown EI, et al. Vacuum-assisted closure: a new method for wound control and treatment: animal studies and basic foundation. Ann Plast Surg 1997;38(6):553–62.

39. Gomoll AH, Lin A, Harris MB. Incisional vacuum-assisted closure therapy. J Orthop Trauma 2006;20(10):705–9.

40. Stannard JP, Robinson JT, Anderson ER, et al. Negative pressure wound therapy to treat hematomas and surgical incisions following high-energy trauma. J Trauma 2006;60(6):1301–6.

41. Stannard JP, Volgas DA, McGwin G III, et al. Incisional negative pressure wound therapy after high-risk lower extremity fractures. J Orthop Trauma 2012;26(1): 37–42.

42. DeCarbo WT, Hyer CF. Negative-pressure wound therapy applied to high-risk surgical incisions. J Foot Ankle Surg 2010;49(3):299–300.

43. Assal M, Stern R. Realignment and extended fusion with use of a medial column screw for midfoot deformities secondary to diabetic neuropathy. J Bone Joint Surg Am 2009;91-A(4):812–20.

44. Hastings MK, Johnson JE, Strube MJ, et al. Progression of foot deformity in Charcot neuropathic osteoarthropathy. J Bone Joint Surg Am 2013;95-A(13):1206–13.

45. Pinzur MS, Schiff AP. Deformity and clinical outcomes following operative of Charcot foot: a new classification with implications for treatment. Foot Ankle Int 2018; 39(3):265–70.

IV. Samuel Merritt – California School of Podiatric Medicine

Clinical Teaching Collaborative Program with California School of Podiatric Medicine and the Samuel Merritt University Motion Analysis Research Center

Tim Dutra, DPM, MS, MHCA[a,b,c,d,e],*, Stephen Hill, BSc, MSc, PhD[f]

KEYWORDS

- Podiatric education • Evidence-based medicine • Biomechanics
- 3D motion analysis • EMG • Kinematics • Kinetics

KEY POINTS

- At Samuel Merritt University (SMU), the California School of Podiatric Medicine (CSPM) collaborates with the Motion Analysis Research Center (MARC) to integrate hands-on quantitative clinical biomechanics research experience into the podiatric medical training program.
- The faculty relates clinical approaches of visual and manual assessment to deeper understand the underlying mechanisms provided by interpretation of quantitative biomechanics data.
- CSPM students enter the MARC with clinical ideas inspired by classes, clinical experience, and study.
- A PhD biomechanist mentors the students to develop their clinical questions, to explore relevant scientific literature, and to formulate research questions to be explored with objective measures.
- Students use a wide variety of motion analysis equipment and techniques and interpret results in the context of original clinical idea and current clinical biomechanical literature.

Funding: Both studies are SMU-internally funded: maximalist shoe study ($24,000 SMU Faculty Support Grant Program) and the ACL and orthotics study ($5000 SMU Seed Grant).
[a] Department of Applied Biomechanics, California School of Podiatric Medicine at Samuel Merritt University, 450 30th Street, Suite 2860, Oakland, CA 94609, USA; [b] Faculty Org, Samuel Merritt University, 2018-2019; [c] Intercollegiate Athletics, University of California, Berkeley, Berkeley, CA, USA; [d] Healthy Athlete Fit Feet Program, Special Olympics, Northern California, Pleasant Hill, CA, USA; [e] Board of Directors, Joint Commission on Sports Medicine & Science; [f] Motion Analysis Research Center, Samuel Merritt University, 400 Hawthorne Avenue, Suite 101, Oakland, CA 94609-3029, USA
* Corresponding author. Department of Applied Biomechanics, California School of Podiatric Medicine at Samuel Merritt University, 450 30th Street, Suite 2860, Oakland, CA 94609.
E-mail address: tdutra@samuelmerritt.edu

INTRODUCTION

At Samuel Merritt University (SMU), the California School of Podiatric Medicine (CSPM) collaborates with the Motion Analysis Research Center (MARC) to integrate hands-on quantitative clinical biomechanics research experiences into the podiatric medical training program. This partnership provides an active learning environment to demonstrate the importance of critical thinking and evidence-based medicine and to demonstrate the role of on-going research in providing patients with the best treatment options available.

The MARC features 2 PhD biomechanists who engage in collaborative research and teaching with faculty and students of Podiatry, Occupational Therapy (OT), Physical Therapy (PT), and the University of California (UC) Berkeley/UC San Francisco Ergonomics Program. The center is well equipped and continually updated with the high-tech tools needed to study movement and collect data (**Fig. 1**). Hardware includes the following:

- Motion Analysis Corporation 12 Kestrel Camera Motion Capture System, featuring Cortex software (Santa Rosa, CA)
- Xsens MVN Analyze: 17 wireless inertial monitoring units: camera-free, full-body 3-dimensional (3D) motion capture (Enschede, Netherlands)
- Qualisys 9-Camera Motion Capture System, featuring Qualisys Tracking Manager software (Gothenburg, Sweden)
- C-Motion Visual 3D, advanced research software for biomechanical analysis of 3D motion capture data (Germantown, MD)
- AMTI Force Platforms (×6) flush-mounted in the floor (Watertown, MA)
- AMTI Instrumented Treadmill with 2 force platforms (Watertown, MA)
- Delsys Trigno Wireless Electromyography (EMG) System (16 channels) (Natick, MA)
- Novel EMED Pressure Mapping System (Munich, Germany)
- Tekscan F-Scan Pressure Mapping System (in-shoes) (South Boston, MA)
- Protokinetics Zeno Gait Walkway (with high-definition webcam) (Havertown, PA)

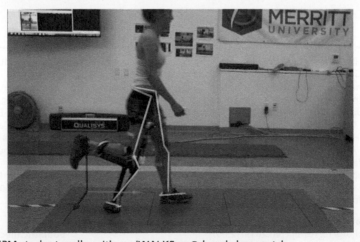

Fig. 1. CSPM student walks with an iWALKFree® hands-less crutch.

- Natus Smart Equitest Balance Manager (sway-referenced floor and visual surround) (San Carlos, CA)
- APDM Mobility Lab Comprehensive Gait and Balance Analysis (Portland, OR)
- Cosmed K5 Wearable Metabolic Testing System (Rome, Italy)
- Lumbar Motion Monitor
- Aretech Zero-G Passive Gait Training System
- Biodex System 4 Pro Isokinetic Dynamometer (**Fig. 2**)

Students gain understanding of the underlying biomechanics of movement by interpreting objective quantitative measurement, as follows:

- Spatiotemporal parameters of gait (step length, step width, toe-out angle, cadence, walking speed, and variability)
- Three-dimensional motion capture (kinematics): whole body, limbs, joints (sagittal/coronal/transverse axes)
- Net joint moments of force (torques)
- Internal joint rotation powers (generation and absorption)
- Surface EMG (muscle activity): phasic bursts, amplitude, frequency
- Pedobarography (plantar pressures of the feet, barefoot or in-shoes)
- Posturography (computerized balance testing)
- Isokinetic strength testing: examining force/velocity relationships of muscle groups
- Cardiopulmonary measures of exertion

These experiences enrich the education of future podiatrists in at least 5 of the following ways:

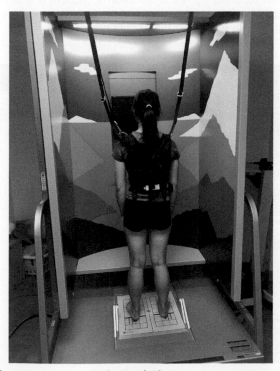

Fig. 2. CSPM student experiences a balance platform.

1. To deepen the knowledge of the mechanisms of human movement, both healthy and pathologic, and interaction of interventions (eg, taping, off-loading, orthotics, assistive devices) by making associations between traditional clinical assessments and quantitative measures.
2. In the future, if they do not have access to quantitative technologies, they may more profoundly understand what they assess clinically, based on previous connections made between the quantitative and visual/manual assessments.
3. To convey the methods and value to the clinical decision process of seeking converging evidence from objective quantitative measurement when available, such as considering referring a patient to a motion analysis laboratory.
4. To prepare these future clinicians to be effective early adopters of clinically valuable quantitative instrumentation as they become available, such as camera systems and wearable sensors; just as the Holter monitor, a battery-operated portable device that records heart activity (electrocardiogram) continuously for 24 to 48 hours or longer, has become a common clinical tool in cardiology.
5. To inspire future clinicians to collaborate with biomechanists and other related professionals in clinical research to contribute to the advancement of Podiatry.
6. At the very least, this exposure to the scientific objective motion analysis will make them better consumers of future clinical research literature (**Fig. 3**).

HISTORICAL PERSPECTIVE

Historically, biomechanics and sports medicine treatment has been based on clinical impressions, patient-reported signs and symptoms, passive and active range of motion (ROM) testing, manual muscle testing, and observations of movements, imaging (radiographs, MRI, and so forth), and differential diagnosis.

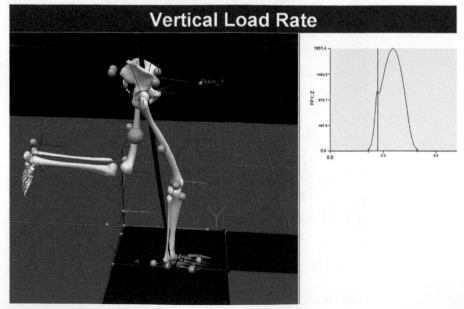

Fig. 3. C-Motion Visual3D Professional analysis software.

It is challenging to control the many interactive variables at play: foot type, foot strike pattern, strength, ROM, shoe gear, inserts/orthotics.

Inclusion/exclusion criteria include the following: consideration of pathologic conditions, deformities, balance, activity, stability, gender, age, size, and medical conditions for possible subject selection for study.

To compare walking with sport-specific movements, the different actions, such as jumping, cutting, backpedaling, lateral movement, as well as balance and muscle activity during specific sports, are compared.

For a motion analysis research opportunity in education and training for CSPM students, students will be engaged in teaching, research, and clinical opportunities in the MARC at different stages of their educational training during their 3 years of classroom education.

TRADITIONAL GAIT EVALUATION (VISUAL)
Taught During Biomechanical Workshop During Second Year

Biomechanical examination
- Weight-bearing versus non-weight-bearing examinations, including hip, knee, ankle, foot, toe ROM and muscle testing, forefoot to rearfoot relationships (varus, valgus, supinatus, elevatus, and so forth); resting calcaneal stance position, neutral calcaneal stance position, knee and leg position; leg length assessment, equinus evaluation.
- Visual gait examination of patient: from head to toe, looking at head position, shoulders, arm swing, hips/pelvis, knee position, tibial position, angle and base of gait, heel contact, propulsion
- Foot type generalizations: pes planus, pes rectus, and pes cavus as reference points
- Shoe generalizations: neutral cushion, motion control, stability; minimalist, maximalist, specialty
- Sport-specific impact: related to sport and surface of activity

To evaluate for the benefit of custom functional orthoses to control motion for activity, the following can be used: posting, top covers, accommodative padding, profile, and fit in specific athletic shoes; troubleshooting and modifications of orthoses.

Pathology-specific orthotics prescription approach to deal with specific biomechanical issues of treatment of the patient.

Podiatrists have developed methods to identify and correct abnormal postures and movement patterns based on foot biomechanics, and we as a profession need to move in this direction.

Podiatric medicine education needs to be based on up-to-date evidence-based scientific principles, and the use of these principles in the biomechanics practice (**Fig. 4**).

TRADITIONAL GAIT EVALUATION (VISUAL)
Taught During Biomechanical Workshop During Second Year

Biomechanical examination: weight bearing versus non-weight-bearing examinations, including hip, knee, ankle, foot, toe ROM and muscle testing, forefoot to rearfoot relationships (varus, valgus, supinatus, elevatus, and so forth); resting calcaneal stance position, neutral calcaneal stance position, knee and leg position; leg length assessment, equinus evaluation.

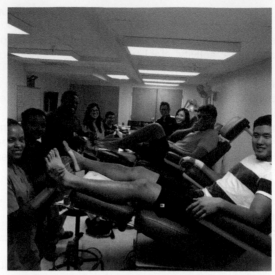

Fig. 4. CSPM students learning low-Dye taping technique.

Visual gait examination of patient: from head to toe, looking at head position, shoulders, arm swing, hips/pelvis, knee position, tibial position, angle and base of gait, heel contact, propulsion.

Foot-type generalizations: pes planus, pes rectus, and pes cavus as reference points.

Shoe generalizations: neutral cushion, motion control, stability; minimalist, maximalist, specialty.

Sport-specific impact: related to sport and surface of activity.

Evaluate for benefit of custom functional orthoses to control motion for activity: posting, top covers, accommodative padding, profile, and fit in specific athletic shoes; trouble-shooting and modifications of orthoses.

A pathology-specific orthotics prescription approach to deal with specific biomechanical issues of the patient: Podiatrists have developed methods to identify and correct abnormal postures and movement patterns based on foot biomechanics. Podiatric medicine education is based on up-to-date evidence-based scientific principles, and the use of biomechanics in practice.

PATH OF CALIFORNIA SCHOOL OF PODIATRIC MEDICINE BIOMECHANICS TRAINING (5 COURSES)

Didactic Coursework in Biomechanics (Biomechanics 1, 2, 3), Clinical Skills

First year: *Biomechanics 1*: basic terminology and concepts of mechanical function, normal development, and dysfunction of the foot, educational model of foot.

Second year: *Biomechanics 2*: common pathologic conditions, pediatric foot, and normal growth; biomechanical evaluation, gait, orthotic principles; emphasis on foot abnormalities, pathologic conditions, and dysfunction. *Biomechanics clinical skills*: workshops on taping, padding, casting, and evaluation of negative cast for orthotics, orthotic prescription and fabrication, gait evaluation, athletic shoe review, biomechanical evaluation, and clinical applications.

Third year: *Biomechanics 3*: Foot pathologic conditions reviewed with emphasis on treatment modalities, gait disturbances, sports medicine, physical medicine and rehabilitation, as well as orthotics and bracing, and surgical biomechanics. *Biomechanics clinical rotation*: emphasis placed on clinical recognition, detection, and conservative treatment, improve proficiency in biomechanical examination, gait, and orthotic troubleshooting; dealing with sports medicine injuries and return to activity guidelines; special physical examination joint and muscle testing.

Motion Analysis Research Center Component of Second-Year Biomechanics Rotation (Since Inception of Motion Analysis Research Center in 2013)

Groups of 8 podiatry students participate in hands-on activities in the MARC, comparing visual qualitative assessment with objective quantitative instrumented gait. First, the biomechanist guides the students to work in pairs to estimate their partner's spatiotemporal parameters of gait: step length, step width, toe-out angle cadence, walking speed, asymmetry; then they compare their estimates to objective measures calculated by the PKMAS software after each student walks along the 8-m Zeno electronic walkway (**Fig. 5**).

Second, the biomechanist guides the group in visually observing the sagittal hip, knee, and ankle angles of the right lower limb during knee points in the gait cycle as 1 person walks across the room (**Fig. 6**).

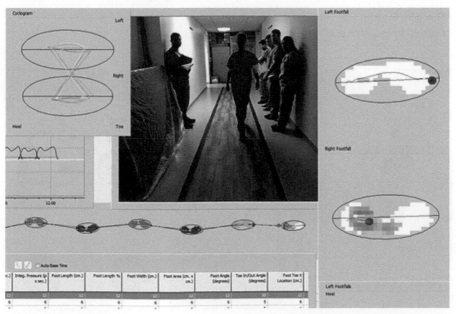

Fig. 5. CSPM students using a Zeno electronic walkway (Protokinetics LLC, Havertown, PA), comparing results to visual estimation of spatiotemporal parameters of gait.

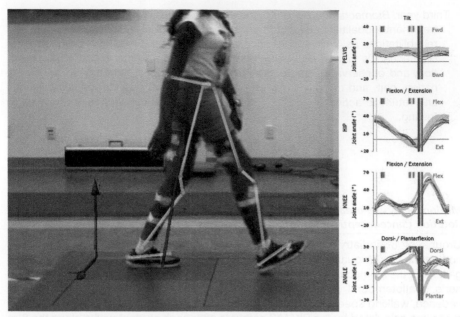

Fig. 6. Video image of participant with knee flexion asymmetry of hemiparetic gait.

Motion Analysis Research Center Component of the Third-Year Biomechanics Rotation (Since July 2017)

Third-year biomechanics rotation is made up of groups of 3 to 5 podiatry students mentored by a PhD biomechanist and a podiatrist (**Fig. 7**).

Creative freedom of clinical research questions.
Guided in feasible pilot project from their ideas.

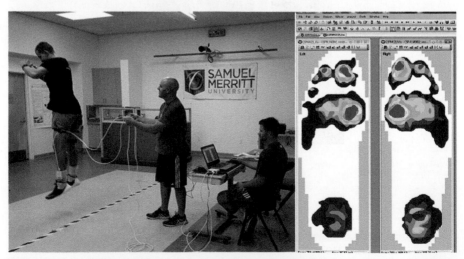

Fig. 7. CSPM third-year students conducting pilot study using Tekscan F-Scan (South Boston, MA) sensors to examine in-shoe foot pressures during jumping.

Review of literature, research questions, design.

Consider relevant methods, technologies.

Taught to instrument participants, setup equipment, collect, analyze, and interpret data.

Present pilot internally: PowerPoint or poster (see **Fig. 7**).

EXAMPLES OF THIRD-YEAR BIOMECHANICS ROTATIONS IN THE MOTION ANALYSIS RESEARCH CENTER

As part of the third-year biomechanics rotation, "pods" of 3 to 5 students work together on a biomechanics project for 3 hours, 1 or 2 times per week for 1 month.

EMG of lower-extremity muscles with iWALK Hands-Free Crutch versus axillary crutches;

Foot pressures in basketball: wood versus pavement playing surface;

Low-dye taping effects on foot and ankle stability and balance.

Limitation: FScan in-shoe foot pressure mapping is good for walking, running, and jumping, but not standing, so standing balance assessed on NATUS Neurocom EquiTest (see **Fig. 2**).

Difficulty recruiting participants in community, including those with clinical conditions.

Training individual students who are working in the MARC during their spare time or within context of a rotation, in contrast to a graduate student who is in the laboratory for a year or more and is more accessible.

Time constraint of 1-month rotation total of 24 hours in the MARC for each 4-student team.

Limits them to pilot studies: team members as participants.

So far, the pilot studies in the third-year biomechanics rotations have not progressed beyond 1 month.

A valuable opportunity for research creativity is provided for each student in this framework.

Podiatry students have opportunities to assist with on-going funded institutional review board (IRB)-approved studies.

Interested students in developing their research ideas into IRB-approved studies are offered mentorship on a case-by-case basis.

SMU INSTITUTIONAL REVIEW BOARD–APPROVED ON-GOING STUDIES

1. *Impact of maximalist running shoes compared to neutral running shoes* funded by a $24,000 SMU Faculty Support Grant Program (PI Cherri Choate, DPM), coinvestigators Stephen Hill, PhD, Andrew Smith, PhD, Timothy Dutra, DPM. Three cohorts, a total of 16 students. Dr Hill mentored the team of podiatry students to collect, analyze, and interpret the overground running data, which they presented at The 2017 Western Foot and Ankle Conference at Anaheim, California. In May 2018, Dr Hill presented further findings of that study at the Gait and Clinical Movement Analysis Society Conference at Indianapolis, Indiana.[2] The team is working on the first journal article from that project with MARC and podiatry faculty and students. The goal is to improve the understanding of the mechanics of different running shoe designs and the potential risks for injuries (**Figs. 8** and **9**).
2. *The role of custom foot orthotics in noncontact anterior cruciate ligament (ACL) injury risk*: $5000 SMU Seed Grant funded study (Drs Stephen Hill and Tim Dutra are co-Primary Investigators) involving healthy female adults with pes planus

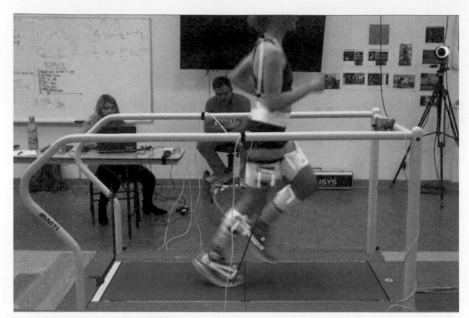

Fig. 8. CSPM student researchers, Hayley Ennis and Kent Cripe, assisting with maximalist shoe research project.

foot type. The ability to establish a direct relationship between a foot orthotic and decreased ACL strain would provide the athletic and medical communities with a preventative course of treatment for a debilitating injury. In the podiatric community, utilization of foot orthoses is a common practice with relatively little risk to athletes. There are long rehabilitation periods associated with a ruptured ACL, not to mention having to undergo a surgical repair. Finding a possible means of preventing, or lessening the frequency of, ACL ruptures would immediately provide a substantial benefit to athletes across the world. Presently, no known studies have examined the effects of custom foot orthotics on

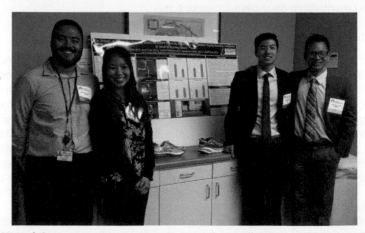

Fig. 9. CSPM students, Kent Cripe, Ivanna Kenwood, Lowell Tong, and Lawrence Chen, presenting a poster at the Kaiser Conference.

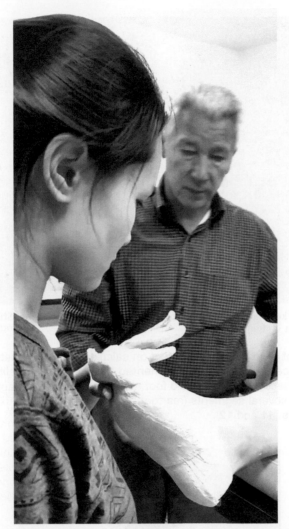

Fig. 10. CSPM student, Yen Tran, casting the foot of a participant under the supervision of Jeff Root, President of the Prescription Foot Orthotic Laboratory Association.

noncontact anterior cruciate ligament risk with knee joint kinematics and kinetics during vertical jumping and lateral "cut" (acute turn) movements during jogging (**Fig. 10**).

3. Oxford foot model interrater reliability. This IRB-approved study explores interrater reliability (2 disciplines: biomechanics research and podiatric clinician) and intrarater reliability (repeated 1 week later) of kinematic tracking marker placement on anatomic landmarks. Two faculty members (Tim Dutra, DPM, and Drew Smith, PhD, Biomechanics) take turns placing markers to identify multiple bony landmarks on the feet of participants, repeating the process 1 week later. Dr Dutra and Dr Hill use the opportunity to expand in depth with the students in visual assessment of gait of the participants while they are in the MARC. This project provides students with opportunities to review surface anatomy with reference to experience gained in the cadaver laboratory. It enforces the

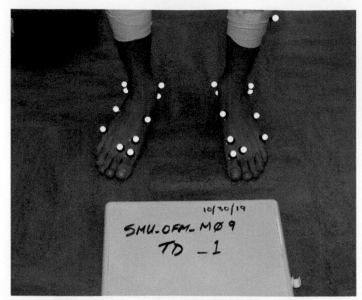

Fig. 11. Foot marker placement on a subject in the Oxford Foot Model Study (markers on posterior heel not visible).

importance of good marker placement on calculating gait kinematics and relates the importance of quantitative instrumented gait analysis to qualitative observational gait assessment. The Oxford foot model was chosen because it separates the foot into several segments (rearfoot, midfoot, forefoot, hallux) of interest to podiatry (**Figs. 11** and **12**).

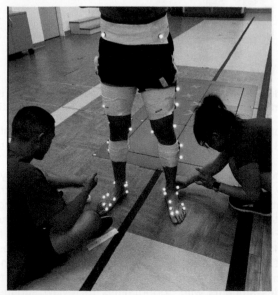

Fig. 12. CSPM students (mentored by Dr Hill) place the markers on the other parts of the lower limbs and pelvis.

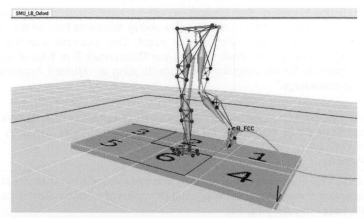

SMU_LB_Oxford

Fig. 13. Software 3D reconstruction of a participant with an Oxford foot model marker set walking over 6 force platforms mounted in the floor of the MARC.

A current CSPM student-driven study is in development: low-dye taping and backpack weight. The study seeks to examine the effect of low-dye taping on plantar pressures on individuals with pes planus feet. Precursory studies describe resulting plantar pressures; however, this study adds the component of external weight with specific weights in a backpack. Students were inspired to explore the effects of external weight on gait, specifically, plantar pressures **(Fig. 13)**.

New Direction for Student Involvement for Research Opportunity

Current pod groups of third-year CSPM students requested to use their month of biomechanics rotation in the MARC on an IRB-approved study (even volunteering their weekends). Modification of the third-year rotation streamlined the research approach for involving interested students and keeping in line with IRB.

Annual Motion Analysis Research Center Symposium

Each year's program includes theme and highlight keynote speakers, presenters in topics of pediatric orthopedics, sports medicine, physical medicine, and rehabilitation Interdisciplinary audience and faculty/students from SMU and the Bay Area are the

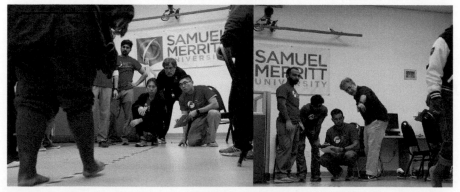

Fig. 14. Dr Dutra and Dr Hill mentoring CSPM students in visual observational gait assessment during the Special Olympics Fit Feet event in the MARC.

primarily audience. Hands-on tutorials and workshops provide interdisciplinary opportunities to participants as well as valuable networking. Students from all disciplines at SMU are encouraged to attend the annual event. One example was the tutorial: Crutches, CAM Walkers, and iWalk: What's the Difference? This tutorial compared 3 different methods for off-weighting patients, looking at different aspects of gait and exercise physiology.[1]

COMMUNITY OUTREACH CLINICAL EXPERIENCES IN COLLABORATION BETWEEN CALIFORNIA SCHOOL OF PODIATRIC MEDICINE AND THE MOTION ANALYSIS RESEARCH CENTER
Special Olympics

Dr Dutra and Dr Hill mentored first-, second-, and third-year CSPM students in gait assessments and recommendations for Special Olympics of Northern California Healthy Athletes Fit Feet Program (**Fig. 14**):

Healthy Athletes Health Fair, SMU MARC, Oakland, March 2, 2019.
Summer Games, UC Davis ARC Pavilion, June 22, 2019.
Floor Hockey Tournament, Alameda County Fair Grounds, Pleasanton, December 7, 2019.
Fall Prevention education in collaboration with Sutter Health, Fall 2017 with balance demonstration in the MARC for community members.
Special case studies in biomechanics: gait analysis in exchange for educational use of data: poststroke gait analysis, hemiparetic gait analysis, posthamstring injury of collegiate football player assessing rehabilitation level, Biodex.
National Biomechanics Day: Hands-on biomechanics demonstrations in the MARC for Alameda High School Sports Medicine class and FACES (Family and Child Education) for the Future Coalition group with the assistance of SMU students from CSPM, PT, and OT, April 10, 2019.

SUMMARY

CSPM + MARC clinical teaching collaborative program provide the opportunity to

- Use qualitative and quantitative biomechanics analysis skills to select and address clinical research questions
- Gain a better understanding of underlying biomechanical mechanisms
- Develop a facility with biomechanical measurement and data interpretation
- Incorporate technological innovations in future clinical practice
- Cultivate research evidence-based clinical practice
- Cultivate approach and understanding of research design and methods for interpreting journal review

FUTURE DIRECTIONS IN EVIDENCE-BASED MEDICINE

Podiatric Biomechanics Fellowship program: being developed in conjunction with the MARC
Special cases community clinic: Special Olympics teams, high school/collegiate/club sports
Interdisciplinary research studies: fall prevention initiatives with PT, OT
Diabetic ulcer/off-loading studies
Preoperative and postoperative surgical planning and follow-up evaluation
Encourage collaboration with prominent alumni interested in biomechanical studies

DISCLOSURE

Dr S. Hill: Member of board who developed American National Standard: ABMSP 001 - 2018, Inserts for Diabetic Footwear American Board of Multiple Specialties in Podiatry for American National Standards Institute (ANSI), Volunteer Faculty Consultant, Special Olympics, Northern California, Healthy Athletes Program: Fit Feet.

ACKNOWLEDGMENTS

The authors acknowledge Drew Smith, PhD, Professor and Director of MARC, and the CSPM students.

REFERENCE

1. Dutra T, Edmunds K, Hill S. Crutches, CAM walkers and iWalk: What's the Difference? Biophysical Answers for Clinical Rx? Workshop presented at: 2nd Annual MARC Symposium: Motion Analysis in Interdisciplinary Healthcare Education and Practice. Oakland, CA, November 4–5, 2016.
2. Hill S, Choate C, Dutra T, et al. Maximalist running shoes compared to neutral running shoes: lower limb kinetics during running. Proceedings of Gait and Clinical Movement Analysis Society Conference. Indianapolis, IN, May 22-25, 2018.

A Comparative Diabetic Foot Wound Measurement Trial Using Wound Tracker Professional Versus Aranz Imaging System and Conventional Ruler Measurement

Alexander M. Reyzelman, DPM[a],*, Shelby McCray, MS, RN[b],
Lacey Beth Peck, DPM[c], Megan Allen, DPM[d], Kris Koelewyn, DPM[e,1]

KEYWORDS

- Wound measurement • Affordable wound measurement system
- IOS application for wound measurement

KEY POINTS

- Wound Tracker Professional wound measurement handheld device can accurately measure wounds.
- iOS application Wound Tracker Professional can track the progression of the wound.
- Wound Tracker Professional is iPhone, iPad, and iPod compatible.
- Wound Tracker Professional is comparable to Aranz medical system and better than acetate tracing in measuring wounds.

INTRODUCTION

In the management of diabetic foot ulcers, the tracking of wound progression is crucial to clinical decision-making. Accurate and reliable wound measurement has been found to be a strong predictor of future healing potential.[1] It provides objective evidence for wound progression and may serve as a useful tool in guiding treatment of patients who may not respond to standard of care.[2] In spite of major advances in wound care technology, wound assessment as well as wound documentation often still relies on rudimentary measures that can be time consuming and inaccurate.

[a] Department of Medicine, California School of Podiatric Medicine at Samuel Merritt University, 3100 Telegraph Avenue, Oakland, CA 94609, USA; [b] Center for Clinical Research, 1107 Mountain Boulevard, Oakland, CA 94611, USA; [c] Oregon Foot Care Centers, 200 N.E. 4th Avenue, Hillsboro, OR 97127, USA; [d] New Mexico VA Healthcare System, 1501 San Pedro SE, Albuquerque, NM 87108, USA; [e] Northport VA Medical Center/Stony Brook University Hospital, 79 Middleville Road, Northport, NY 11768, USA
[1] Present address: 1019 Fort Salonga Road Suite 10 #199, Northport, NY 11768.
* Corresponding author. 2299 Post Street Suite 205, San Francisco, CA 94115.
E-mail address: areyzelman@samuelmerritt.edu

Clin Podiatr Med Surg 37 (2020) 279–285
https://doi.org/10.1016/j.cpm.2019.12.012
0891-8422/20/© 2020 Elsevier Inc. All rights reserved.

Today, the most widely used measuring device used by practitioners is a handheld ruler or probe to measure the length, depth, and width of a wound.[3] Despite its cost-effectiveness and ease of use, this method of wound measurement models the wound as a rectangle and thus has been found to be inaccurate for irregularly shaped wounds.[4] The Kundin Gauge similarly uses a set of 3 paper rulers set at orthogonal angles to measure wound dimensions. Another most commonly used method to measure a wound is the tracing method, wherein a wound is outlined using a sterile two-ply transparent sheet. The top layer is then placed over a measuring grid and the area calculated with a planimeter. This method, although low cost, entails wound contact and additional labor for instance, averaging multiple measurements for accuracy.[5] Other more advanced measures require additional setup and equipment; stereophotogrammetry uses a camera and a computer to create a 3-dimensional (3D) wound construct, whereas software-based tracing of digital photographs to calculate wound area. Most recently, there has been development of devices such as the Aranz Silhouette, which couples Personal Digital Assistance (PDA) technology with laser-assisted digital photography for 3D measurement.[3] Despite Aranz becoming the new gold standard in wound measurement for clinical research, it is not an affordable system in most of the private practice and clinical settings.

Thomas and Wysocki[6] state that the selection of a wound assessment tool should entail consideration for cost, time, and purpose of measurement. Morison and Bjellerup[7,8] even make the argument that tracking percent change in wound size, rather than its absolute dimensions, is sufficient in most clinical settings. In this light, it becomes apparent that widespread adoption of any advanced wound assessment tool would first necessitate product portability, cost-effectiveness, and ease of use. With the Wound Tracker Professional (WTP) the aim was to develop and test a tool that can meet the abovementioned criteria while providing accurate and consistent wound measurements.

Today, more than 85 million iPhones and 34 million iPads have been sold worldwide by Apple. Apple offers unique software that is exclusive to Apple products.[9] The iOS operating system is user friendly and allows individuals to gain access to more than 500,000 plus applications available at the Apple App Store. Currently, more than 80 applications have been developed specifically for health care professionals. Doctors are now able to hold textbooks, drug formulas, medical calculators, and more by downloading an app. With this advancement in technology, they offer on the go access to information that could help improve patient care. Apple products have become ubiquitous among the general population, which makes for a consistent platform for the WTP application.[10] In addition, the Aranz Silhouette is currently mostly being used for research purposes, whereas the WTP is meant to be used in a clinical-based setting.

The investigators of this study used an application available for iOS, which brings wound measurement and tracking right to the palm of the hand. This innovative application is the first of its kind to be unveiled for the iOS platform. WTP is an application available for the iOS platform, which allows the user to take a picture of a wound, measure the area, and keep track of the patient's wound progress. The application combines advanced measurement of a given wound area with the ability to view previous measurements and photographs right at bedside. This application eliminates hardware commitment and allows virtually everyone with a device running iOS to use the application.

The sole purpose of the study is to determine the accuracy of the WTP application. The data collected within the application were compared with the manual data collected (disposable transparent film tracing) and wound measurements done by the Aranz Silhouette. The authors' hypothesis is that the iOS application (WTP) is more accurate than conventional measurement of wounds (disposable transparent film tracing) and as accurate as digital measurement (Aranz Silhouette).

METHODS
Inclusion and Exclusion Criteria

The Institutional Research Board at Samuel Merritt University approved this study and all participants provided informed consent before performing study procedures. For this prospective pilot study, data from 20 patients with a documented pedal wound were collected between March 2015 and October 2015. Patients included in the trial were 18 years or older and with a pedal wound on the plantar surface of the foot. Patients were excluded if they had any unstable medical condition that would cause the study to be detrimental to the subject as judged by the Principal Investigator or if they are bedridden or are unable to come to the clinic. Patients were selected from the patient population of the private practice office of the principle investigator.

At the initial visit, the research assistants considered inclusion and exclusion criteria and ascertained the willingness of the patient to participate in the clinical study. The subject's participation in this study was completely voluntary, and subjects were free to decline or withdraw at any point. Participation in the study did not affect or change patients' clinical care or treatment regimen in any manner, because routine measurement of wound size is already standard of care for treating neuropathic wounds. Patients were only subjected to 2 extra measurements of the pedal wound if they agreed to be apart of the study.

Data Collection

Following enrollment, patients were selected at random to participate, which served to control variables such as age, sex, socioeconomic status, occupation, and coexisting unidentified factors. No patient identifiers were used in the collection of data (application allowed for fictitious names, numbers, or initials). First the patient's pedal wound was measured with disposable transparent film dressing and the Aranz Silhouette, which served as the accepted gold standard. The same pedal wound was then measured using the IOS application (WTP) on an IPod Touch device. The measurements obtained were the pedal wound length and width. From those values, the Aranz Silhouette and WTP calculated the area of the wound in square centimeters. In order to avoid intraobserver error, one person was performing the measurements throughout the course of the trial.

RESULTS

Data from 20 consented patients with a documented pedal wound were obtained. The minimum, maximum, median, and mean values were calculated in standard fashion. Area is represented in square centimeters and is calculated using software algorithms for both the Aranz and WTP systems. The total wound area for the acetate tracing is also represented in square centimeters and calculated using simple area = length x width formula. The values of importance include the following: (1) the average length (in centimeter) measured by the disposable transparent film dressing, the Aranz Silhouette, and WTP were 1.61, 1.64, and 1.56, respectively; (2) the average width (in centimeter) measured by the disposable transparent film dressing, the Aranz Silhouette, and WTP were 1.22, 1.16, and 1.26, respectively; and (3) the average area (in square centimeter) measured by the disposable transparent film dressing, the Aranz Silhouette, and WTP were 2.37, 1.72, and 1.69, respectively. Each method of measurement was then compared with the current gold standard, Aranz Silhouette, for accuracy. The P values for comparing the paired differences from the gold standard or the paired WTP versus tracing differences were computed using the nonparametric Wilcoxon signed rank test. As shown in **Table 1**, the P value when comparing WTP area to ARANZ area is not statistically significant, but the difference between tracing area and ARANZ area is statistically significant. The mean percentage difference signifies the average difference in measurement between either the WTP or acetate compared with the gold-standard ARANZ measurement. This statistical was calculated using the following formula: MPD = (mean difference/gold standard mean) x 100. On average, WTP measured the exact same wound area as ARANZ by a difference of −1.7%. Comparatively, the acetate tracings versus the gold standard were significantly off by an average of 38.3%. **Table 1** summarizes these results.

DISCUSSION

Since the 2003 Sheehan landmark article[1] on wound healing prediction, the wound care industry has evolved into a multibillion dollar business. Various pharmaceutical companies have spent millions to develop products to facilitate or augment wound healing. The foundation of wound healing begins with the treating physician and his or her ability to recognize and address factors that may be contributing to slow progression of healing. Regardless of the type of wound being treated, recognition of the progression of the wound gives the treating physician or a wound care provider the ability to modify treatment.

Progression of the wound has been historically monitored with documentation, which includes depth, length, and width of a given wound along with a thorough description of the wound base, peri-wound skin, drainage, and odor. With the advent of digital photography and Electronic Medical Records, the visual progression of a wound has gained popularity, as pictures of a particular patient's wound can be uploaded to the patient's chart for comparison.

With the advancement of technology and arrival of PDA the wound care industry had major developments. The Aranz Silhouette incorporated PDA technology along with digital photography and a laser-assisted system, which allows for 3D measurement and tracking of wounds size. This system is currently being used in a research setting due to cost and hardware commitment, whereas the average wound care professionals do not use it. The need for a more portable, widely available, less expensive tool is still lacking. As previously mentioned, the ability to keep track of a patient's wound essentially governs treatment and their treatment regimen. The inherent problem with manual measurements is that no matter what the shape of the wound is, the area that is being calculated is that of a rectangle. However, most of the wounds are irregularly shaped and require a different method of measurement that more accurately assesses the area. There is a need for a device that can measure and store wound measurements in a patient's record that is user friendly and easily accessible such as the Aranz Silhouette and now WTP.

Wound Tracker Professional

WTP is a new iOS application that is compatible with the iPhone, iPad, and iPod touch. It allows users to take a picture of a wound, which can then be used to track the patient's wound until it is completely healed. The application also takes a fast measurement of the wound and then calculates the area of the wound. By the use of this application, an individual is able to visually track the progression of the wound. One of the best features of the application is its functionality. Initially when the application

Table 1
Statistical analysis of 3 separate parameters and their comparison with each other

Parameter	Variable	Min	Median	Mean	Max	P Value[a]	Mean % Difference
Area (cm²)	Aranz—gold standard	0.30	1.10	*1.72*	5.60	—	—
Area (cm²)	Tracing	0.40	1.47	2.37	8.06	—	—
Area (cm²)	WTP	0.20	1.20	1.69	6.40	—	—
Comparison							
Area (cm²)	Tracing difference from Aranz	−0.28	0.37	0.66	3.96	0.0002	38.3%
Area (cm²)	WTP difference from Aranz	−1.90	0.00	−0.03	0.80	0.7480	−1.7%
Area (cm²)	Trace difference from WTP	−4.00	−0.30	−0.69	0.08	0.0000	−40.0%

Parameter	Variable	Min	Median	Mean	Max	P Value[a]	Mean
Length (cm)	Aranz—gold standard	0.80	1.40	*1.64*	3.20	—	—
Length (cm)	Tracing	0.80	1.40	1.61	3.10	—	—
Length (cm)	WT	0.50	1.40	1.56	3.10	—	—
Comparison							
Length (cm)	Tracing difference from Aranz	−0.30	0.00	−0.03	0.20	0.3486	−1.8%
Length (cm)	WT difference from Aranz	−0.60	−0.10	−0.08	0.10	0.0181	−4.9%
Length (cm)	Trace difference from WT	−0.60	0.00	−0.05	0.20	0.3282	−3.0%

Parameter	Variable	Min	Median	Mean	Max	P Value[a]	Mean
Width (cm)	Aranz—gold standard	0.40	1.10	*1.16*	2.30	—	—
Width (cm)	Tracing	0.50	1.10	1.22	2.60	—	—
Width (cm)	WT	0.30	1.20	1.26	2.60	—	—
Comparison							
Width (cm)	Tracing difference from Aranz	−0.30	0.00	0.07	1.20	0.7720	5.6%
Width (cm)	WT difference from Aranz	−0.40	0.05	0.10	1.20	0.2789	8.7%
Width (cm)	Trace difference from WT	−0.50	0.00	0.04	0.30	0.2676	3.0%

[a] Nonparametric Wilcoxon signed rank P value.

is launched the user has to register and set up a password to ensure patient privacy. Following registration, the user has the ability to either add a new patient or choose a patient from the database. New measurements can be made for each patient at subsequent visits. When taking a picture of a wound the user has to include a presized reference box, included and printable within the program, to ensure accuracy and eliminate the need to estimate camera-to-wound distance at each measurement. The user then follows screen instructions to align the reference box and outline the wound. Once this is done, the area of the wound along with the maximum vertical and horizontal distance is calculated. The user has the ability to add comments and save the measurement.

The user can review previous measurements and pictures of the patient's wound individually or the subsequent measurements can be graphed and viewed for better comparison. The application also allows the user to generate a PDF patient report that includes a graph of the patient's wound progression along with the pictures of the patient's wound at each measurement, which the user may print, upload, or email.

New measurements can be made for each patient at subsequent visits or anytime desired.

There are several advantages to using this application when compared with other similar concepts such as the Aranz Silhouette and a few are discussed here. As previously mentioned, the paramount advantage is that there are no hardware commitments. The application works on the iPhone, iPad, and iPod Touch devices, which are widely available and owned by most practitioners or staff. This allows the application to be used by many practitioners and virtually anyone with the previously mentioned devices. In addition, the ability to share measurements and pictures of a patient's wound instantly via email allows anyone to relay information to the treating physician. Users also may choose to email the reports to an electronic medical record program or print the summary and save to a patient's file. Moreover, the application is user friendly with on-screen instructions, a detailed instruction manual, and video embedded into the application itself.

In summary, this pilot trial using WTP has demonstrated to be as accurate as the Aranz medical system with a mean percentage difference in wound area of only 1.7% (a P-value of 0.7480). Comparatively, the traditional method of acetate tracing or simple length versus width to obtain a total wound area value varies from the gold standard by almost 40% (a P-value of 0.0002).

WTP offers the user the ability to organize the history and see the progression of a patient's wound. The lack of hardware commitment, ease of use, and the ability to share or email information into the patient's medical chart add to the advantages of this application. With an affordable price tag, the application is an enticing way to improve patient care without a substantial risk.

Limitations

The small number of patients included in the authors' dataset limited this study. Additional subjects may have increased the power of this study. One way that we tried to avoid interobserver reliability was to use only 1 iPod Touch device with the loaded WTP application for data collection and 1 practitioner who collected data on all 20 patients. The authors realize that this might not be practical for all clinical based settings, but for their study they desired to maintain consistency while gathering data.

DISCLOSURE

The authors have nothing to disclose.

REFERENCES

1. Sheehan P, Jones P, Giurini JM, et al. Percent change in wound area of diabetic foot ulcers over a 4-week period is a robust predictor of complete healing in a 12-week prospective trial. Diabetes Care 2003;26:1879–82.
2. Lait ME, Smith LN. Wound management: a literature review. J ClinNurs 1998; 7:11–7.
3. Kieser DC, Hammond C. Leading wound care technology: the ARANZ medical silhouette. Adv Skin WoundCare 2011;24:68–70.
4. Jessup RL. What is the best method for assessing the rate of wound healing? A comparison of 3 mathematical formulas. Adv Skin WoundCare 2006;19:138–45.
5. Springle S, Nemeth M, Gajjala A. Interactive design and testing of a hand held non contact wound measurement device. J TissueViability 2012;21:17–26.
6. Thomas A, Wysocki A. The healing wound; a comparison of three clinically useful methods of measurement. Decubitus 1990;3:18–25.

7. Bjellerup M. Cost benefit requirements in the management of wounds. WoundMa-
   nagement 1996;1:7–8.
8. Morison M. Pressure sores: assessing the wound. Professional Nurse; 1989.
   p. 532–5.
9. Tsukayama H. "How many iphones has apple sold?" Washington Post. The Washington Post 2012. Web. 28 July 2014.
10. Payne KF, Wharrad H, Watts K. Smartphone and medical related app use among
    medical students and junior doctors in the United Kingdom: a regional survey.
    BMC Med Inform DecisMak 2012;12:121.

V. Kent State University College of Podiatric Medicine

Intrinsic Fixation of the Tibial Sesamoid in First Metatarsophalangeal Joint Arthrodesis: A Cadaveric Study

Emily E. Zulauf, DPM[a],*, James C. Connors, DPM[b],
Allan M. Boike, DPM[c], Mark A. Hardy, DPM[b]

KEYWORDS

• Tibial sesamoid • First MTP joint • Fusion • Hallux rigidus

KEY POINTS

• First metatarsophalangeal joint arthrodesis with tibial sesamoid fixation is an economical alternative to plating.

• Locking plate construct for first metatarsophalangeal joint arthrodesis demonstrates higher maximum load to failure than K-wire fixation.

• Fixation of tibial sesamoid neutralizes lever arm of the flexor hallucis brevis.

INTRODUCTION

Hallux rigidus, the most common form of arthritis in the foot, is a degenerative condition of the first metatarsophalangeal (MTP) joint. It is defined by a progressive loss of joint space leading to decreased motion, increased pain, and alteration of gait mechanics.[1]

MTP joint arthrodesis is a well-documented salvage procedure for treatment of a variety of deformities, including hallux abducto valgus, osteoarthritis, end-stage hallux rigidus, hallux varus, failed first MTP joint arthroplasty, and degenerative joint disease associated with trauma.[2–7] Interestingly, reported fusion rates are higher with a diagnosis of hallux rigidus versus hallux valgus.[3] Various fixation methods have been described to fuse the first MTP joint, including single or multiple Kirschner wires (K-wires), Steinmann pins, staples, neutralization plates, compression screws, or a combination of the above.[3,5,6,8,9] A systematic review of early weight-bearing after arthrodesis of the first MTP joint describes use of fixation constructs in 17 studies

[a] Grant Medical Center, 323 East Town Street, First Floor, Suite 100, Columbus, OH 43215, USA;
[b] Division of Surgery and Biomechanics, Kent State University College of Podiatric Medicine, 6000 Rockside Woods Boulevard, Independence, OH 44131, USA; [c] Kent State University College of Podiatric Medicine, 6000 Rockside Woods Boulevard, Independence, OH 44131, USA
* Corresponding author.
E-mail address: Emily.zulauf@gmail.com

Clin Podiatr Med Surg 37 (2020) 287–293
https://doi.org/10.1016/j.cpm.2019.12.003
0891-8422/20/© 2019 Elsevier Inc. All rights reserved.

podiatric.theclinics.com

of 898 arthrodesis procedures. Approximate utilization of each fixation construct was as follows: 34.08% plate fixation, 21.38% crossed compression screws, 13.92% single compression screw, 9.69% catgut suture, 9.35% K-wire or cerclage wire, 7.80% staples, 3.79% with no internal fixation.[10] Advances in internal fixation, such as the advent of anatomic plating, have led to use of more expensive constructs.[6] In 2008, a cost comparison study revealed a significant difference in hardware cost of crossed screws versus dorsal plate for first MTP joint arthrodesis with no difference in fusion rate.[5] A retrospective study of 138 feet showed no significant difference in time to fusion or rate of fusion between static and locked plating constructs, with or without a lag screw.[9] Storts and Camasta[6] evaluated incidence of union with buried K-wire fixation versus crossed screw construct with immediate weight-bearing and found their buried K-wire technique to yield a fusion rate of 98%.[6] Rate of fusion reported for first MTP joint arthrodesis with various constructs ranges between 77% and 100%.[4,7,8,11]

The function of the first MTP joint sesamoid complex is to stabilize the first ray and increase mechanical advantage of the flexor hallucis brevis tendon (FHB). The sesamoids, embedded in FHB tendons, adductor hallucis, and abductor hallucis, dynamically stabilize the MTP joint by resisting dorsiflexion of the hallux.[12] The sesamoids increase the lever arm of the FHB to augment push-off strength at the MTP joint, propelling the foot off the ground in the last moment of push-off phase of gait. Most fixation constructs ignore the inherent mechanical advantage of the sesamoid complex by not incorporating the sesamoids.

To the authors' knowledge, no study has examined strength of an augmented construct with tibial sesamoid fixation for treatment of hallux rigidus. The authors find that sesamoid fixation effectively neutralizes the lever arm of the FHB, providing comparable fusion rates, decreasing surgical costs, and allowing early weight-bearing in the appropriate patient population. This study aimed to investigate the strength of the first MTP joint sesamoid fixation combined with traditional arthrodesis methods in the first MTP.

MATERIAL AND METHODS

Fifteen fresh frozen cadaveric limbs were divided into 3 groups (A, B, and C) with 5 limbs per group. A linear dorsomedial incision with first MTP joint dissection was performed on each limb. A single surgeon (A.B.) performed all 15 procedures to reduce variability in technique (**Figs. 1** and **2**). The experimental groups were fixated as follows:

Group A: Four K-wires oriented in a locking construct across the joint (n = 5)

Group B: Four K-wires oriented in a locking construct across the joint with 1 K-wire bisecting the tibial sesamoid, oriented perpendicular to weight-bearing surface from dorsal to plantar (n = 5)

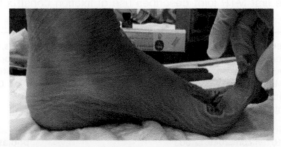

Fig. 1. Clinical dorsiflexion obtained before K-wire fixation.

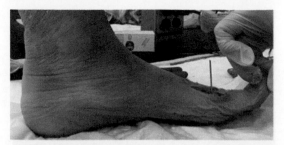

Fig. 2. Clinical dorsiflexion obtained following K-wire fixation of the tibial sesamoid.

Group C: Locking plate fixation with interfragmentary screw (n = 5)

Fixation was verified with anteroposterior and lateral plain film radiography (**Figs. 3** and **4**). Next, each specimen was resected at the level of the first metatarsal-cuneiform joint. Care was taken to maintain pertinent soft tissue structures, including the FHB tendon. Each specimen was embedded with Bondo adhesive into a PVC pipe construct before biomechanical testing. An MTS 858 Mini Bionix material testing system (MTS Systems, Eden Prairie, MN, USA) was used to axially load each specimen at

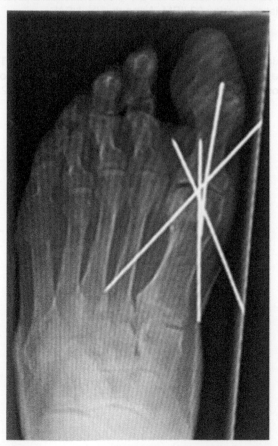

Fig. 3. AP radiograph of group A configuration with 4 K-wires oriented in a locking construct.

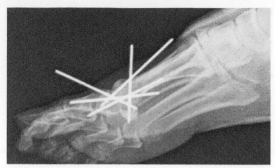

Fig. 4. Lateral radiograph of group B construct with 1 K-wire bisecting the tibial sesamoid.

the distal first MTP joint, simulating propulsion (90 N, rate of 5 Hz) until clinical failure (**Fig. 5**). Clinical failure was defined as failure of the limb/specimen, hardware failure, or gapping of the joint. Maximum load of the cell achieved. Load at time of clinical failure was recorded.

Descriptive and inferential statistics were performed using a 1-way analysis of variance with a significance point established at $P<.05$. Statistical analysis was performed using SPSS Statistics, version 22 (IBM, Armonk, NY, USA).

RESULTS

The average maximum load at the point of clinical failure is shown in **Table 1**. Group C demonstrated the greatest maximum load before failure at 153.5 N, followed by group B at 110.1 N. Group A had the lowest maximum load to failure at 72.9 N.

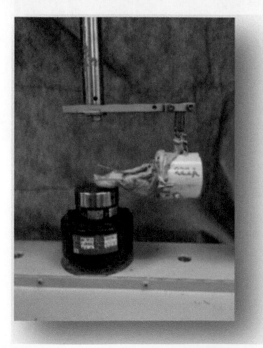

Fig. 5. A material testing system loading specimen at distal first MTP joint simulation propulsion.

Table 1		
Average maximum load at point of clinical failure		
Group	Average Maximum Load (N)	Standard Deviation (N)
A	72.9	9.5 ± 4.76
B	110.1	9.3 ± 5.4
C	153.5	18.9 ± 11.5

Data from 1 specimen in group A was excluded for improper loading in the cell because of its large size relative to other specimens. One specimen from each group B and group C were excluded because of multiple data points on the MTS load displacement curve, and no visual failure point was observed.

The authors' study showed no statistically significant difference in average maximum load between groups A and B. The mean maximum load before failure was 72.9 N in group A and 110.1 N in group B. The addition of 1 K-wire to fixate the tibial sesamoid increased fixation strength by 28.8 N on average. Mean maximal load to failure for the locking plate was 153.5 N, which was significant ($P = .004$) compared with groups A and B (see **Table 1**). The locking plate demonstrated the highest average maximum load to failure and thus was the strongest fixation method tested (**Fig. 6**).

DISCUSSION

Arthrodesis of the first MTP joint is the gold standard for treating patients with osteoarthritis. It has been documented to provide excellent functional outcomes and high patient satisfaction.[11] Traditional postoperative management recommends 4 to 6 weeks of non-weight-bearing.[13] However, instances where non-weight-bearing increases risk of complications, such as falls and deep vein thrombosis, warrant efforts to begin patients ambulating faster postop. Immediate weight-bearing postoperatively should decrease incidence of disuse atrophy, osteopenia, and prolonged recovery associated with immobilization and non-weight-bearing.[7,14]

Reported use of robust fixation constructs, such as anatomic plates and screws allowing for earlier weight-bearing, is increasingly noted in the literature.[4] However, increased strength of fixation is not without consequence. Anatomic plate and screw fixation contributes to the exorbitant amount of health care costs.[5,15] A level II cost

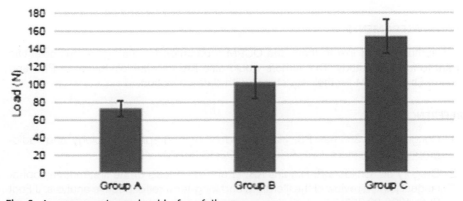

Fig. 6. Average maximum load before failure.

analysis by Rothermel and colleagues[16] in 2019 compared the cost of synthetic hydrogel implants against the cost of an average first MTP joint fusion plate and associated screws. The implant was quoted to cost $3825 and the plate construct was quoted to cost roughly $1660. In contrast, K-wires are estimated to cost less than $10.[6] Storts and Camasta[6] describe their technique with buried K-wires to allow for more points of fixation across the fusion site, increasing incidence of fusion. Surgeon's use of materials in the operating room is under increased scrutiny as the emphasis on cost containment increases. Surgeons face increased pressure to eliminate unnecessary procedural costs. The authors' fixation construct for first MTP joint arthrodesis offers an economical alternative to conventional plating with the added benefit of early weight-bearing.

There are several limitations to the present study. Cadaveric studies cannot possibly replicate functional relationships of weight-bearing human biomechanics. Loss of soft tissue and muscular stability limits the biomechanical testing model as well. True gait mechanics was not simulated because the first MTP joint was isolated and axially loaded to failure. As such, the tested construct was prone to failure at the adhesive Bondo-specimen interface. In future studies, the authors recommend direct screw fixation to the cadaveric bone to decrease motion at the adhesive interface. The authors' sample size was small (n=15), increasing variability and rendering the results less reliable. Three specimens were removed from analysis: 1 sample was too large to be tested uniformly at the same point as the other specimens. The authors recommend selecting cadaveric specimens that are similar in size and weight to allow for better comparison and to decrease variability with load cell setup and testing.

Based on the findings of this study, addition of a single K-wire into the tibial sesamoid provides increased strength to the first MTP joint arthrodesis construct. Sesamoid fixation in first MTP joint fusion has been described as adding inherent increase in stability.[6] By neutralizing the lever arm of the FHB with sesamoid fixation, this study showed a 28.8-N increase in load to failure. According to Campbell and colleagues,[17] approximately 25% of an individual's body weight can be supported at the first MTP joint. The simple K-wire technique may allow patients to withstand greater force and therefore bear weight earlier in the postoperative course.[14] The same study also highlights the added benefit of overall cost savings with use of K-wires.

DISCLOSURE

The authors have nothing to disclose.

ACKNOWLEDGMENTS

The authors would like to thank the OCPM foundation for their generous scientific grant to fund this study. The authors would also like to thank Jill Kawalec, PhD and Duane Ehredt, DPM for their assistance with data collection.

REFERENCES

1. Coughlin MJ, Shurnas PS. Hallux rigidus: demographics, etiology and radiographic assessment. Foot Ankle Int 2003;10(24):731–43.

2. Gregory JL, Childers R, Higgins KR, et al. Arthrodesis of the first metatarsophalangeal joint: a review of the literature and long-term retrospective analysis. J Foot Surg 1990;29:369–74.

3. Korim MT, Mahadevan D, Ghosh A, et al. Effect of joint pathology, surface preparation and fixation methods on union frequency after first metatarsophalangeal joint arthrodesis: a systematic review of the English literature. Foot Ankle Surg 2017;23(3):189–94.

4. Berlet GC, Hyer CF, Glover JP. A retrospective review of immediate weight bearing after first metatarsophalangeal joint arthrodesis. Foot Ankle Spec 2008; 1:24–8.

5. Hyer CF, Glover JP, Berlet GC, et al. Cost comparison of crossed screws versus dorsal plate construct for first metatarsophalangeal joint arthrodesis. J Foot Ankle Surg 2008;47:13–8.

6. Storts EC, Camasta CA. Immediate weightbearing of first metatarsophalangeal joint fusion comparing buried crossed Kirschner wires versus crossing screws: does incorporating the sesamoids into the fusion contribute to higher incidence of bony union? J Foot Ankle Surg 2016;55(3):562–6.

7. Abben KW, Sorensen MD, Waverly BJ. Immediate weightbearing after first metatarsophalangeal joint arthrodesis with screw and locking plate fixation: a short-term review. J Foot Ankle Surg 2018;57(4):771–5.

8. Roukis TS. Nonunion after arthrodesis of the first metatarsal-phalangeal joint: a systematic review. J Foot Ankle Surg 2011;50(6):710–3.

9. Hyer CF, Scott RT, Swiatek M. A retrospective comparison of four plate constructs for first metatarsophalangeal joint fusion: static plate, static plate with lag screw, locked plate, and locked plate with lag screw. J Foot Ankle Surg 2012;51(3): 285–7.

10. Crowell A, Van JC, Meyr AJ. Early weightbearing after arthrodesis of the first metatarsal-medial cuneiform joint: a systematic review of the incidence of nonunion. J Foot Ankle Surg 2018;57(6):1204–6.

11. DeSandis B, Pino A, Levine DS, et al. Functional outcomes following first metatarsophalangeal arthrodesis. Foot Ankle Int 2016;37(7):715–21.

12. McCormick J, Anderson RB. Turf toe: anatomy, diagnosis, and treatment. Sports Health 2010;2(6):487–94.

13. Yu GV, Shook JE. Arthrodesis of the first metatarsophalangeal joint. In: Banks AS, Downey MS, Martin DE, et al, editors. Comprehensive textbook of foot surgery. 3rd edition. Philadelphia: Lippincott; 2001. p. 581–607.

14. Mah CD, Banks AS. Immediate weight bearing following first metatarsophalangeal joint fusion with Kirschner wire fixation. J Foot Ankle Surg 2009;48(1):3–8.

15. Tejwani NC, Guerado E. Improving fixation of the osteoporotic fracture: the role of locked plating. J Orthop Trauma 2011;25(Suppl 2):S56–60.

16. Rothermel SD, King JL, Tupinio M, et al. Cost comparison of synthetic hydrogel implant and first metatarsophalangeal joint arthrodesis. Foot Ankle Spec 2019. https://doi.org/10.1177/1938640019850617.

17. Campbell B, Schimoler P, Belagaje S, et al. Weight-bearing recommendations after first metatarsophalangeal joint arthrodesis fixation: a biomechanical comparison. J Orthop Surg Res 2017;12(1):1–6.

Acute Deltoid Ligament Repair in Ankle Fractures
Five-year Follow-up

Mark A. Hardy, DPM[a], James C. Connors, DPM[a],*,
Emily E. Zulauf, DPM[b], Michael A. Coyer, DPM[c]

KEYWORDS

- Ankle instability • Bimalleolar equivalent • Deltoid injury • Medial malleolar complex
- Syndesmotic injury

KEY POINTS

- Acute deltoid repair in unstable bimalleolar equivalent ankle fractures restores medial ankle stability and anatomic alignment.
- The direct repair of the deep deltoid leads to high patient satisfaction and return to normal activity levels.
- The use of suture tape and anchors provide long-lasting stability without significant complications due to internal hardware.

INTRODUCTION

The deltoid ligament is understood to be one of the primary ligamentous stabilizers of the ankle joint.[1–3] Anatomically, the deltoid ligament is composed of a fan-shaped, vertically oriented superficial layer traversing 2 joints and a horizontal deep layer spanning the ankle joint.[4] The superficial layer consists of the tibionavicular, tibiocalcaneal, and posterior tibiotalar ligaments and primarily resists eversion of the hindfoot.[5] The deep deltoid layer includes the deep anterior tibiotalar and deep posterior tibiotalar ligaments and its transverse orientation limits external rotation of the talus.[4,5] The densely packed parallel collagen bundles of the deltoid ligament combined with fiber-rich interlacing collagen

[a] Division of Surgery and Biomechanics, Kent State University College of Podiatric Medicine, 6000 Rockside Woods Boulevard, Independence, OH 44131, USA; [b] Grant Medical Center, 323 East Town Street, First Floor, Suite 100, Columbus, OH 43215, USA; [c] Private Practice, Orange County Foot and Ankle Surgeon, 16405 Sand Canyon Avenue, Suite 270, Irvine, CA 92618, USA
* Corresponding author.
E-mail address: charcotforecastinginitiative@gmail.com

Clin Podiatr Med Surg 37 (2020) 295–304
https://doi.org/10.1016/j.cpm.2019.12.004
0891-8422/20/© 2020 Elsevier Inc. All rights reserved.

allows for multidirectional tensile strength—counteracting talar valgus tilting, anterior translation, and external rotation throughout the gait cycle.[3,4,6–8] The structural importance and role of the deltoid ligament make its repair in acute ruptures highly contested.[9,10] It has been previously thought that rigid fixation of the distal tibiofibular syndesmosis and associated fracture fixation allow for ligamentous healing negating the need for primary deltoid repair.[1] The basis of this idea, however, is rooted in historical unstandardized studies with small sample sizes and poor patient follow-up.[2]

In many cases of acute ankle fractures, surgeons address syndesmotic instability but have a high threshold to primarily repair the deltoid. Even with syndesmotic fixation, deltoid insufficiency may lead to overcompensation at the distal tibiofibular articulation, resulting in ankle instability.[11] Primary repair of the deltoid ligament with concomitant fibular fracture fixation ultimately may aid in prevention of malalignment leading to posttraumatic ankle arthrosis.[12,13] Ligamentous or osseous instability of the medial ankle complex can significantly alter joint biomechanics and accelerate tibiotalar cartilage damage.[5] With the joint destructive nature of end stage arthritic ankle joint procedural options, the use of a preemptive primary medial deltoid repair is warranted.[2]

PATIENTS AND METHODS

A retrospective review of all patients undergoing acute medial deltoid ligament repair by the senior author (MH) occurring between January 1, 2005, and December 31, 2014, was completed; 24 total patients were identified meeting the inclusion criteria of sustaining either a bimalleolar or trimalleolar equivalent ankle fracture with medial clear space widening on stress radiographs (**Fig. 1**). Fourteen patients

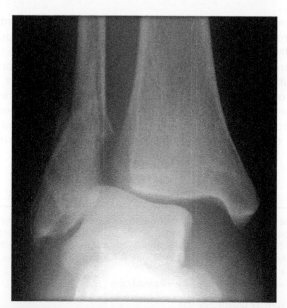

Fig. 1. Displaced and unstable bimalleolar equivalent ankle fracture with obvious medial deltoid injury.

were interested in participating in the study. This cohort was found to have 10 Weber B and 4 Weber C fractures with 11 bimalleolar and 3 trimalleolar equivalent variants. Concurrent syndesmotic fixation was performed in 9 cases of suture endobutton. Four medial malleolus avulsion fractures were identified preoperatively, with 1 patient requiring excision of the fragment secondary to fragment instability and infolding of the deltoid ligament. Patients were contacted by phone and completed a modified patient outcome satisfaction survey that measured functional return to activity and pain relief postoperatively. At last clinical follow-up, all records indicated satisfactory healing and patients were discharged from care with no restrictions.

Pain and success scores were described using an ordinal scale with medians and interquartile ranges. The paired Wilcoxon signed rank test was used to test significance between preoperative and postoperative pain scores. Categorical variables were described using counts and percentages. Data analysis was completed using R software (version 3.0.2, Vienna, Austria).

All surgical procedures were performed by the senior author (MH). Patients were placed on the operating table in supine position and underwent general anesthesia. A standard thigh tourniquet was utilized. A linear 3-cm incision was placed over the medial malleolus for inspection of the deltoid ligament. The medial talar dome and medial ankle gutter were exposed to verify infolding or attenuation of the deep

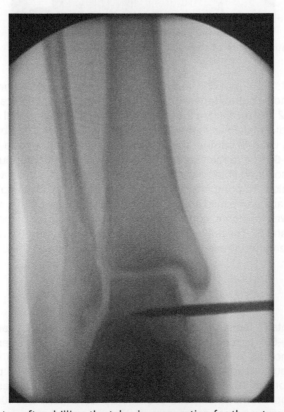

Fig. 2. A 4.5-mm tap after drilling the talus in preparation for the suture tape placement.

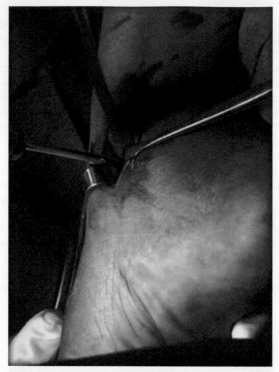

Fig. 3. Intraoperative picture of the talar drill hole being taped.

deltoid ligament. A 2.7-mm drill bit and 4.5-mm tap were utilized per manufacturer guidelines to place a suture tape with bioabsorbable anchor into the medial body of the talus (**Figs. 2** and **3**). Next, a 2.5-mm drill bit was utilized to drill an oblique hole through the medial malleolus in the direction of the deep deltoid fibers. A microsuture passer was used to capture the previously placed suture tape from the suture anchor (**Figs. 4–6**). The repair was then secured with a hemostat but not tensioned because the associated fibular fracture and any syndesmotic injury were addressed in standard fashion. To complete the medial repair, the ankle was placed in neutral in the sagittal plane and a mild supinatory force was applied at the subtalar joint as the suture arm was tensioned and secured to the medial cortex of the tibia via suture button (**Figs. 7** and **8**). The ankle then was placed through range of motion and verified to be stable under stress fluoroscopy with restoration of the distal tibiofibular overlap.

RESULTS

Fourteen patients (7 female and 7 male) with mean age of 42 years (interquartile range [IQR] 17–68) agreed to participate in the study and were followed on average 70.6 months (5.9 years). Of these patients, the median subjective preoperative pain scale was 9 (IQR 5–10) out of 10, which improved postoperatively to 1 (IQR 0–5) out of 10. The median decrease in pain score was 8 (IQR 3–10). The median improvement of pain score was 90.7 (IQR 65–100) out of 100, and the median score rating the overall success of the procedure was 91.1

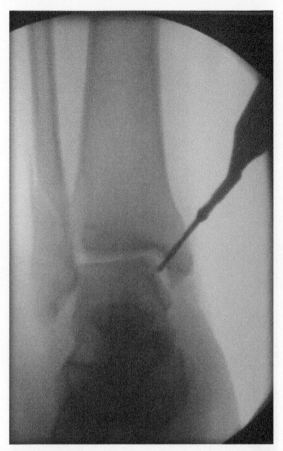

Fig. 4. Intraoperative image of the microsuture passer through the medial malleolus drill hole to shuttle the suture tape providing stability to the deep deltoid.

(IQR 60–100) out of 100. The median satisfaction score for return to normal activity was 93 (IQR 70–100) out of 100 and higher-demand activities 88 (IQR 60–100) out of 100. The overall return to function capacity measured 85.5 (IQR 33–100). One -patient had lateral hardware removed without disruption of the medial repair. Two patients complained of medial swelling with activity but reported no activity limitations.

No reports of infections or wound complications were reported within the study population. No patients required revision or medial hardware removal.

DISCUSSION

Stability of the medial ankle complex is due largely to the intact deltoid ligament.[1–3] Incidence of medial deltoid ligament injury in acute ankle fractures may be higher than historically reported. Hintermann and colleagues[12] found 40% of their 288 ankle fractures to have deltoid ligament injury and advocated that primary operative repair should be considered given that satisfactory results have been achieved. Shen and colleagues[1] primarily repaired 34 acute

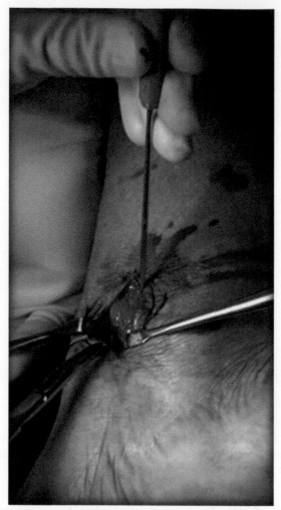

Fig. 5. Intraoperative image of the microsuture passer shuttling the suture tape through the medial malleolus.

deltoid ligament ruptures associated with ankle fractures and found persistent medial ankle instability after fracture fixation prior to ligamentous repair. Stress evaluation of the medial ankle after fracture fixation should be used to assess for residual instability—if identified, primary repair should be considered.[2,9,12,14–16]

Acute ankle fractures with suspected deep deltoid ligament interruption classically are addressed via fracture fixation and syndesmotic repair, indirectly allowing the deltoid to statically heal.[17] Reduction of the syndesmosis has been found to be significantly associated with functional outcomes.[18] More recent publications, however, have reported superior outcomes in patients undergoing deltoid repair after acute trauma. Hsu and colleagues[14] treated 14 National Football League players with medial deltoid avulsion injuries who were able

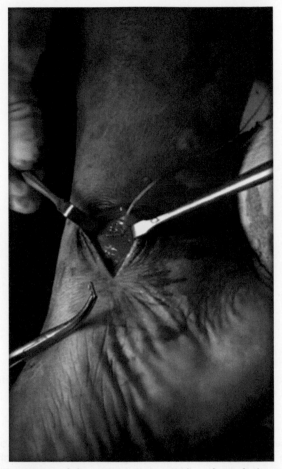

Fig. 6. Intraoperative image of the suture tape extending through the medial malleolus.

to return to sport at the same level within 6 months. No complications or postoperative instability was reported. Yu and colleagues[15] repaired 131 ruptured deltoid ligaments associated with ankle fracture injuries and reported that primary repair can prevent ankle stabilization-related complications. Rigby and Scott[2] recommend débridement and primary repair of the deltoid after fracture fixation to avoid changes in tension after fracture reduction. Dabash and colleagues[10] conducted a systematic review of outcomes of acute ankle fractures with deltoid ligament reconstruction (137 ankles) versus without deltoid ligament reconstruction (144 ankles). They reported no significant difference in the AOFAS ankle scores between the 2 groups; however, the repair group showed a statistically significant lower complication rate. The investigators suggest that the higher malreduction rate in the nonrepair group may have influenced this result.[10]

The authors reported long-term patient satisfaction outcomes after acute deltoid repair with suture anchors in the setting of ankle fractures with more than 5-years follow-up, on average. The results confirm patients were able to return to normal function utilizing the described deltoid repair technique. Patients were exceedingly

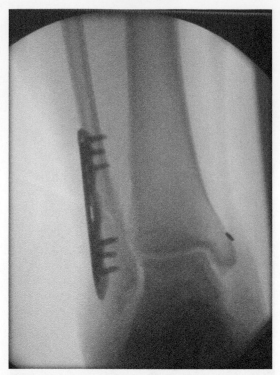

Fig. 7. Intraoperative anterior-posterior fluoroscopic image of the completed deltoid suture button placement after fibular fixation.

satisfied with their outcome and rated their ability to return to normal activity at 93%. Long-term follow-up validates the longevity of the repair technique. The authors believe direct visualization of the deltoid ligament rupture and its repair allow for more precise anatomic restoration of joint congruity than relying on syndesmotic fixation alone. As with any surgical procedure, the possibility for future complications remains; however, within the population, minimal negative outcomes were reported. No secondary or revision procedures were required. No patients reported hardware irritation necessitating removal.

Limitations of this study include its retrospective nature, reliance on patient participation, and small patient population. Additionally, the deltoid ligament rarely is an isolated repair and concomitant procedures were performed at the time of repair. Radiographic imaging at the time of survey completion would have been beneficial but was not obtained. Results of this investigation could be used in development of future randomized controlled trials or prospective cohort studies in a larger population. Ultimately, randomized controlled trials are necessary to establish standards of care for deltoid ligament injury, but more recent literature suggests benefits of deltoid repair outweigh long-term risks.

DISCLOSURE

The authors have nothing to disclose.

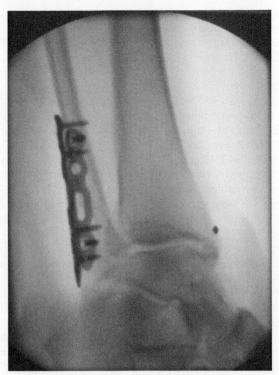

Fig. 8. Intraoperative oblique fluoroscopic image of the completed deltoid suture button placement after fibular fixation.

REFERENCES

1. Shen JJ, Gao YB, Huang JF, et al. Suture anchors for primary deltoid ligament repair associated with acute ankle fractures. Acta Orthop Belg 2019;85(3): 387–91.
2. Rigby RB, Scott RT. Role for primary repair of deltoid ligament complex in ankle frctures. Clin Podiatr Med Surg 2018;35(2):183–97.
3. Rein S, Hagert E, Schneiders W, et al. Histological analysis of the structural composition of ankle ligaments. Foot Ankle Int 2015;36(2):211–24.
4. Panchani PN, Chappell TM, Moore GD, et al. Anatomic study of the deltoid ligament of the ankle. Foot Ankle Int 2018;35(9):916–21.
5. Kusnezov NA, Eisenstein ED, Diab N, et al. Medial malleolar fractures and associated deltoid ligament disruptions: current management controversies. Orthopedics 2017;40(2):e216–22.
6. Savage-Elliot I, Murawski CD, Smyth NA, et al. The deltoid ligament: an in-depth review of anatomy, function and treatment strategies. Knee Surg Sports Traumatol Arthrosc 2013;21(6):1316–27.
7. Hajewski CJ, Duchman K, Goetz J, et al. Anatomic syndesmotic and deltoid ligament reconstruction with flexible implants: a technique description. Iowa Orthop J 2019;39(1):21–7.
8. Massri-Pugin J, Lubberts B, Vopat BG, et al. Role of the deltoid ligament in syndesmotic instability. Foot Ankle Int 2018;39(5):598–603.

9. van den Bekerom MP, Mutsaerts EL, Dijk van CN. Evaluation of the integrity of the deltoid ligament in supination external rotation ankle fractures: a systematic review of the literature. Arch Orthop Trauma Surg 2009;129:227–35.

10. Dabash S, Elabd A, Potter E, et al. Adding deltoid ligament repair in ankle fracture treatment: is it necessary? A systematic review. Foot Ankle Surg 2018. https://doi.org/10.1016/j.fas.2018.11.001.

11. Boden SD, Labropoulos PA, McCowin P, et al. Mechanical considerations for the syndesmosis screw. A cadaver study. J Bone Joint Surg Am 1989;71:1548–55.

12. Hintermann B, Knupp M, Pagenstert G. Deltoid ligament injuries: diagnosis and management. Foot Ankle Clin 2006;11(3):625–37.

13. Femino JE, Vaseenon T, Phisitkul P, et al. Varus external rotation stress test for radiographic detection of deep deltoid ligament disruption with and without syndesmotic disruption: a cadaveric study. Foot Ankle Int 2013;34(2):251–60.

14. Hsu AR, Lareau CR, Anderson RB. Repair of acute superficial deltoid complex avulsion during ankle fracture fixation in national football league players. Foot Ankle Int 2015;36:1272–8.

15. Yu GR, Zhang MZ, Aiyer A, et al. Repair of the acute deltoid ligament complex rupture associated with ankle fractures: a multicenter clinical study. J Foot Ankle Surg 2015;54(2):198–202.

16. Wang X, Zhang C, Yin JW, et al. Treatment of medial malleolus or pure deltoid ligament injury in patients with supination-external rotation type IV ankle fractures. Orthop Surg 2017;9(1):42–8.

17. Gardner MJ, Demetrakopoulos D, Briggs SM, et al. Malreduction of the tibiofibular syndesmosis in ankle fractures. Foot Ankle Int 2006;27:788–92.

18. Weening B, Bhandari M. Predictors of functional outcome following transsyndesmotic screw fixation of ankle fractures. J Orthop Trauma 2005;19:102–8.

VI. New York College of Podiatric Medicine

The Impact of Vitamin D Levels in Foot and Ankle Surgery

Matrona Giakoumis, DPM[a,b],*

KEYWORDS

- Vitamin D • Hypovitaminosis D • Foot and ankle • Nonunion • Bone healing

KEY POINTS

- Vitamin D deficiency and insufficiency, also referred to as hypovitaminosis D, is a major global health problem.
- Given the importance of vitamin D in the maintenance of bone health, osteotomy and arthrodesis surgery outcomes, osteointegration, and implant longevity, the focus of this article is to provide an up-to-date review of the literature with a focus on the role of vitamin D in foot and ankle surgery.
- Although there is a paucity of high-level studies, recent publications recommend screening and treatment of hypovitaminosis D.
- A potential study design is proposed that may provide high-level data regarding hypovitaminosis D and bone healing success.

INTRODUCTION

Vitamin D deficiency and insufficiency, also referred to as hypovitaminosis D, is a major global health problem. It is estimated to affect more than 1 billion people worldwide and affects third world countries as well as industrialized countries.[1,2] If one was to perform a PubMed search using the keyword vitamin D, the search would return about 82,517 hits. Scrolling through the results, it quickly becomes evident that vitamin D is associated with or has implications in a multitude of nonmusculoskeletal health and musculoskeletal health outcomes. These outcomes range from periodontitis, child dental caries, preeclampsia, cancer, autoimmune disorders, cardiovascular disorders, infectious diseases, neurologic disorders, diabetes, wound healing complications, and a multitude of bone disorders.

Causes and risk factors of hypovitaminosis D include inadequate sun exposure, sunscreen use, darker skin pigmentation, increasing latitudes, increasing age, obesity, use

[a] Department of Surgical Sciences, New York College of Podiatric Medicine, 53 East 124th Street, New York, NY 10035, USA; [b] The Podiatry Institute, Decatur, GA, USA
* New York College of Podiatric Medicine, 53 East 124th Street, New York, NY 10035.
E-mail address: mgiakoumis@nycpm.edu

Clin Podiatr Med Surg 37 (2020) 305–315
https://doi.org/10.1016/j.cpm.2019.12.009
podiatric.theclinics.com

of certain medications, genetic and acquired disorders, gastrointestinal malabsorption syndromes, malnutrition, liver dysfunction, and renal insufficiency (**Table 1**).[2–6]

From a skeletal standpoint, vitamin D supports a variety of tissues, is vital to bone growth and maintenance, and prevents sequelae of deficiency including rickets in children and osteomalacia in adults.[7,8] Although the literature is limited, hypovitaminosis D has been associated with delays in fracture healing and increased frequency of nonunion.[9–11] Hypovitaminosis D can also result in muscle weakness, atrophy, arthralgia, and can bring out neurologic changes affecting postoperative rehabilitation.[12–16]

It has even been reported that the single most cost-effective way to reduce global mortality is to double world mean vitamin D levels.[17] Given the importance of vitamin D in the maintenance of bone health, osteotomy and arthrodesis surgery outcomes, osteointegration, and implant longevity, the focus of this article is to provide an up-to-date review of the literature with a focus on the role of vitamin D in foot and ankle surgery.

VITAMIN D METABOLISM

Vitamin D, a regulatory hormone, consists of two different compounds: ergocalciferol (vitamin D_2) and cholecalciferol (vitamin D_3) (**Fig. 1**). Vitamin D_2 and D_3 are inactive precursors, derived from plant sterols and from skin exposed to sunlight, respectively. Vitamin D is also available through fortified foods, such as milk and oral supplements. Absorption of calcium from the intestine is dependent on active vitamin D, 1,25(OH) 2D, which is dependent on an intact liver and kidney. When vitamin D is produced cutaneously, the process is initiated by the conversion of 7-dehydrocholesterol to vitamin D_3 by ultraviolet B radiation.

Regardless of the source, D_2 and D_3 must undergo a two-step enzymatic hydroxylation. They are first converted by D-25-hydroxylase in the liver to 25-hydroxyvitamin D (25-OH D, also known as calcidiol). They are then further converted in the renal proximal tubule by 25-hydroxyvitamin D 1-α-hydroxylase to the active form of the vitamin, 1,25(OH)2D (calcitriol). Production is under homeostatic control because it is regulated by circulating parathyroid hormone concentrations.

Once activated, vitamin D acts through common vitamin D receptors. These vitamin D receptors are located on nearly all cells throughout the human body, further highlighting the integral role vitamin D plays in cellular function.[2,18–23] Homeostatic interaction between parathyroid hormone, calcium, and phosphate regulate the production of 1,25-dihydroxyvitamin D.[24,25] Mobilization of calcium from bone by vitamin D occurs via receptor activator of nuclear factor-κB ligand induced osteoclastogenesis. When vitamin D levels are low, the absorption of calcium and phosphate in the intestine is

Table 1
Causes and risk factors leading to hypovitaminosis D

Inadequate Sun Exposure	Use of Certain Medications
Sunscreen use	Genetic and acquired disorders
Darker skin pigmentation	Gastrointestinal malabsorption syndrome
Increasing latitudes	Malnutrition
Increasing age	Liver dysfunction
Obesity	Renal insufficiency

Data from Refs.[2–6]

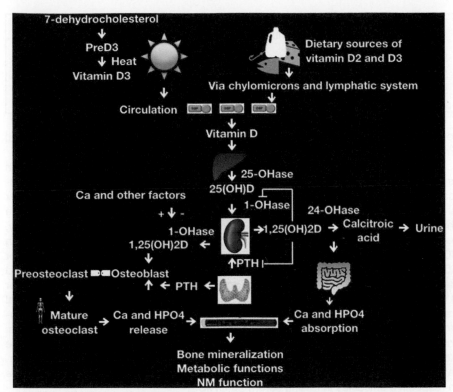

Fig. 1. Metabolism pathway of vitamin D from cholecalciferol, synthesized in skin by activation of ultraviolet B, along with dietary and supplement ingestion of cholecalciferol and ergocalciferol. The various different metabolic effects of 1,25(OH)2D on bone metabolism, calcium, and phosphorus is also illustrated.

decreased by half. To maintain the normal calcium-to-phosphate ratio, parathyroid hormone production is increased, resulting in increased osteoclastic resorption and secondary hyperparathyroidism.[26]

VITAMIN D LEVELS, BONE HEALTH, AND MANAGEMENT OF VITAMIN D

Calcidiol, 25-OH D is the major circulating metabolite of vitamin D in the bloodstream and has a half-life of 15 days.[27] It is the standard measure of vitamin D status and serves as a biomarker for exposure, when repleting levels, and when screening for deficiency. However, no standard measurement exists, and different laboratories report values as either nanograms per milliliter (ng/mL) or nanomoles per liter (nmol/L) (1 ng/mL = 2.5 nmol/L),[28] with variability also existing among the defined values of the normal range. To establish what level of vitamin D is necessary for optimum health, the Institute of Medicine reviewed available data to define deficiency, inadequacy, adequacy, and toxicity. Toxicity is rare, but may manifest as nausea, vomiting, diarrhea, headache, lethargy, muscle and joint pain, increased urination, kidney stones, or cardiac arrhythmia.[29] The Endocrine Society (**Table 2**) defines vitamin D deficiency as less than 20 ng/mL or less than 50 nmol/L. Vitamin D insufficiency is defined as 21 to 29 ng/mL or 52.5 to 72.5 nmol/L. Anything greater than 30 ng/mL or 75 nmol/L is considered sufficient. However, these definitions according

Table 2		
Serum 25-hydroxyvitamin D [25(OH)D] concentrations and status		
ng/mL	nmol/L	Status
<20	<50	Deficient
21–29	52.5–72.5	Insufficient
≥30	≥75	Sufficient

to the Institute of Medicine, the Mayo Clinic and the American Association of Clinical Endocrinologists are all different, leading to a lack of consensus.

The recommended daily allowance in healthy individuals to maintain bone health and normal calcium metabolism has been established by the Endocrine Society clinical practice guideline.[30] The recommended dietary intake is based on age and sex and is reported in international units (IUs) and micrograms (mcg) and on the premise that the individual is receiving minimal sun exposure (**Table 3**). In cases of deficiency, recommended supplementation is intended to reach and maintain levels greater than 30 ng/mL.[31] For individuals aged 1 to 18, the recommended daily dose is 2000 IU or 50,000 IU once a week for 6 weeks followed by a maintenance dose of 600 to 1000 IU daily. For adults, the recommended daily dose is 6000 IU or 50,000 IU once a week for 8 weeks followed by a daily maintenance dose of 1500 to 2000 IU. There are special cases, for instance, patients with increased body mass index, malabsorption syndromes or who take medications that affect vitamin D metabolism. For these cases, the recommended daily dose is 6,000 IU to 10, 000 IU, followed by a maintenance dose of 3,000-6,000 IU/day. Although the interchangeable use of D_2 or D_3 supplementation has been reported to be acceptable,[31] other studies have pointed to a difference in respective efficacies in raising serum 25(OH)D.[32–35]

Tripkovic and colleagues[35] performed a systematic review and meta-analysis comparing vitamin D_2 and vitamin D_3 supplementation in raising serum 25-hydroxyvitamin D status. Their initial electronic database search resulted in 3030 potential articles. After assessment for possible inclusion, 10 studies were included for systematic review, and 7 studies were included for meta-analysis. The conclusion of the meta-analysis indicated that vitamin D_3 was more efficacious at raising serum 25(OH)D concentrations. The authors did, however, recommend further research to examine the metabolic pathways involved and to examine the effects of age, sex, and ethnicity. In terms of ethical consideration, one should also note that vitamin D_3 is not suitable for vegans and therefore not all patients.

Another area of interest relates to the role of simultaneous supplementation of calcium with Vitamin D. Burt and colleagues[36] undertook a randomized clinical trial to assess the effect of daily vitamin D at high doses on volumetric bone density and bone strength on 311 healthy adults. If concomitant dietary intake of calcium was less than 1200 mg per day, daily calcium supplementation was provided. Participants

Table 3	
Recommended vitamin D supplementation dose based on age and deficient serum 25(OH)D concentration	
Age	Supplement Dose
1–18 y of age	2000 IU daily or 50,000 IU once a week for 6 wk Maintenance: 400–1000 IU
>18 y of age	6000 IU daily or 50,000 IU once a week for 8 wk Maintenance: 1500–2000 IU

were randomized into the pilot cohort or the main cohort. The main cohort included three different interventions (400 IU vitamin D_3 daily, 4000 IU vitamin D_3 daily, or 10,000 IU vitamin D_3 daily) and the participants were followed for 3 years. Statistically significant lower radial bone mineral density was observed in participants receiving 4000 or 10,000 IU per day and tibial bone mineral density was significantly lower with the 10,000 IU group, indicating that higher doses are not more beneficial.

Therefore, is supplementing with vitamin D alone enough? According to a Cochrane review looking at vitamin D supplementation and risk of hip fractures in institutionalized elderly patients, vitamin D had to be given along with calcium to be effective in the prevention fractures.[4]

ANIMAL STUDIES

Several animal studies have been published investigating vitamin D and healing. Bhamb and colleagues[37] used a rat posterolateral fusion model to study the effect of modulating dietary vitamin D on general bone health. The authors were able to show that increasing vitamin D during the perioperative period improved femoral strength, stiffness, and density.[37] Other animal studies studied the contents of fracture callous makeup and have established an increased accumulation of vitamin D[38,39] at the site.

IMPLICATIONS IN FOOT AND ANKLE SURGERY

In 2017, a five-member panel sponsored by the American College of Foot and Ankle Surgeons published a clinical consensus statement on perioperative management using a modified Delphi method. Regarding the routine preoperative assessment of vitamin D levels on all foot and ankle arthrodesis procedures, the panel was unable to reach a consensus.[40] They did, however, comment that measurement of the preoperative vitamin D level may elucidate an unrecognized piece of the patient's overall health.

In fact, preoperative screening of patients undergoing foot or ankle surgery may find that hypovitaminosis D is present in most individuals. Based on a systematic review and meta-analysis by Sprague and colleagues,[41] the weighted pooled prevalence of hypovitaminosis D was 70%. The primary analysis included 54 studies (involving primarily hip fractures) and the secondary analysis included meeting abstracts. The authors did not find any trends in prevalence of hypovitaminosis D by latitude or continent. Another interesting observation with important clinical involvement is the emerging evidence of large acute decreases in serum vitamin D levels after a fracture. This raises a good question: "does hypovitaminosis D in fracture patients represent pathology that needs to be corrected to improve fracture healing outcomes, or are the observed low serum levels a normal acute phase reaction in the setting of a 70% baseline prevalence of hypovitaminosis D in the general nonfracture population?"

Despite the literature, which points to high rates of vitamin D deficiency in orthopedic trauma patients,[42–47] there is a paucity of high-level studies regarding foot and ankle surgery and how vitamin D deficiency affects outcomes. When performing a search on National Institutes of Health's Clinical Trials on "bone fracture" and "vitamin D" (eliminating hip fractures), 56 results populated. When further searched for "bone healing" or to include "foot and ankle," there were no results for prospective or randomized control trials. However, a few level 3 and level 4 studies were identified, including studies looking at prevalence of hypovitaminosis D in foot and ankle trauma patients, and elective surgical procedures.

Smith and colleagues[48] were interested in identifying the prevalence of vitamin D deficiency in patients presenting with foot or ankle fractures. They compared the prevalence in this group of patients with the prevalence of vitamin D deficiency in a group of patients presenting with ankle sprain only (low-energy injury). Forty-seven percent (35 of 75) of patients were found to have vitamin D insufficiency and 13% (10 of 75) were vitamin D sufficient. Compared with the ankle sprain group, the level of vitamin D was significantly lower in the fracture group ($P = .02$).

A recent multicenter study[49] prospectively obtained serum vitamin D levels in 577 consecutive patients undergoing elective foot and ankle surgery during the preadmission assessment. The authors found that 21.7% of the patients were grossly deficient, 31.9% were deficient, 28.9% were insufficient, and only 17.5% were considered within the normal range. Nonwhite ethnicity and winter months had statistically lower vitamin D levels.

A case series published by Brinker and colleagues[10] involving 37 patients from a larger series of 683 consecutive patients with a nonunion identified underlying endocrine and metabolic dysfunction in 31 of the 37 patients (84%). Twenty-five of those 31 patients had a vitamin D abnormality and supplementation alone resulted in successful union in 8 of the 31 patients.

Another case-control retrospective study published by Moore and colleagues[50] compared 29 patients with nonunion following elective foot and ankle reconstruction with a control group of 29 patients with successful union. They assessed for the prevalence of modifiable risk factors including body mass index, use of tobacco, diagnosis of diabetes mellitus, vitamin D abnormality, thyroid dysfunction, and parathyroid disease. A statistically significant ($P<.05$) difference was identified between the two groups for endocrine and metabolic disease. The presence of vitamin D deficiency was significantly associated with nonunion ($P = .002$) and a patient was 8.1 times more likely to develop a nonunion if there was a diagnosis of vitamin D deficiency or insufficiency (95% confidence interval, 1.996–32.787).

Michelson and Charlson[51] prospectively obtained the vitamin D status of 81 patients undergoing a major ankle, hindfoot, or midfoot arthrodesis. They were also interested in specifically looking at this group, which resides at a latitude of 44.5° N given that latitude higher than 30° N has been found to be a risk factor for hypovitaminosis D.[52] Of the 81 patients, 44% (36 of 81) were already on vitamin D supplementation by the primary care provider. Of the patients tested, 67% (54 of 81) were found to have low levels. After supplementation, about 56% of the retested group corrected to normal. The authors did note an overall fusion rate of 85%, regardless of testing status or vitamin D status. Further elucidation regarding vitamin D status and bone healing would have been of interest, particularly looking at union rate between normal and abnormal vitamin D levels or even abnormal and corrected levels before surgery. Unfortunately, because of study size, this was not possible.

POTENTIAL STUDY DESIGN

To study the relationship between hypovitaminosis D and nonunion, a prospective multicenter randomized control trial is proposed. In the proposed trial, patients presenting for elective foot and/or ankle arthrodesis procedures will have their serum 25(OH) level drawn preoperatively. If results are found to be deficient or insufficient, patients will be randomly allocated into one of two study groups or the control group. Study group A would receive vitamin D supplementation alone, study group B would receive vitamin D and calcium, and the control group would receive a placebo.

The proposed trial inclusion criteria would be as follows: adult subjects 18 years of age or older, a minimum of 1 year of follow-up data from the surgery date, and surgical reconstruction of foot and/or foot pathology by joint arthrodesis. The exclusion criteria should be as follows: incomplete records or incomplete follow-up, previous nonunion, previous infection, peripheral neuropathy, Charcot neuroarthropathy, hepatic dysfunction, renal dysfunction, and vitamin D resistance caused by X-linked hypophosphatemic rickets.

Supplementation of vitamin D would be based on the Endocrine Society Clinical Practice Guidelines. For the vitamin D and calcium supplement group, adults younger than 50 years of age or less would be given 1000 mg of daily calcium and adults older than the age of 50 would be given 1200 mg of daily calcium. Michelson and Charlson[51] supplemented individuals with hypovitaminosis D with 50,000 IU D_2 three times a week for 2 to 3 months; however, only about 56% of those patients normalized. Based on previous reports,[35] D_3 instead of D_2 may be more effective at normalizing levels and would be used in this study. Because of a lack of consensus regarding the optimal dose regimen, the suggested supplement doses may prove to be inadequate. Vitamin D levels should be rechecked every 4 weeks for normalization. Once blood levels normalize, patient would be placed on a maintenance dose and proceed to surgery.

The primary aim of the proposed study is to measure time to union and union rate within the two treatment groups and control group. The secondary outcome measures will assess the influence of age, sex, race, type of arthrodesis surgery, presence of diabetes mellitus, presence of peripheral neuropathy, and tobacco use.

Plain film radiographs would be obtained at regular intervals to look for signs of bone healing. Successful arthrodesis would be defined as consolidation of the arthrodesis site and obliteration of joint space on more than one radiographic view. Clinically, patients should have an absence of warmth and swelling to the surgical site. Nonunion would be determined by the guidelines set forth by the Food and Drug Administration and is defined as lack of progressive signs of healing for 3 months or lack of any trabeculation for 9 months.

Potential benefits for the proposed research would be to further establish the benefit of preoperative screening for hypovitaminosis D in patients undergoing elective foot and/or ankle arthrodesis procedures. The study would also help to establish if vitamin D_3 alone is sufficient to normalize hypovitaminosis D or if concomitant supplementation of calcium is necessary.

SUMMARY

It is well established that hypovitaminosis D is present among patients with foot and ankle injuries and those undergoing elective foot and ankle procedures. The consequences of hypovitaminosis D are recognized in the literature along with the potential musculoskeletal and nonmusculoskeletal benefits of sufficient levels. Several recently published articles recommend that surgeons do their due diligence and diagnose and treat patients with hypovitaminosis D, particularly preoperatively.[53,54]

Given the observation of a decrease in vitamin D levels during fusion healing[37] and during the early phase of fractured bone healing,[55] does a new "sufficient" level for patients undergoing foot and ankle fracture repair or arthrodesis procedures need to be established? Does the preoperative threshold of what is considered sufficient need to be higher? Should the standard of care of preoperative patients include checking 25(OH) levels and normalizing them before elective procedures?

Childs and colleagues[56] performed a cost benefit analysis of supplementing all fracture patients with vitamin D and calcium during the first 8 weeks of fracture healing. They report an annual nonunion mean of 3.9% of the fracture repair group at their facility, which results in about $78,030 in treatment costs per year. They found that if all patients were supplemented, despite the cost of supplementing, there would be a net savings of $65,866.

Therefore, until further evidence-based medicine refutes it, preoperative screening and treatment of hypovitaminosis D may benefit patients from a healing standpoint but may also prove to provide a socioeconomic gain.

DISCLOSURE

Consultant for Medartis and Royal Biologics.

REFERENCES

1. Holick MF. The vitamin D deficiency pandemic: approaches for diagnosis, treatment and prevention. Rev Endocr Metab Disord 2017;18(2):153–65.
2. Holick MF. Vitamin D deficiency. N Engl J Med 2007;357:266–81.
3. Patton CM, Powell AP, Patel AA. Vitamin D in orthopaedics. J Am Acad Orthop Surg 2012;20(3):1123–9.
4. Avenell A, Gillespie WJ, Gillespie LD, et al. Vitamin D and vitamin D analogues for preventing fractures associated with involutional and post-menopausal osteoporosis. Cochrane Database Syst Rev 2009;(2):CD000227.
5. Sullivan SS, Rosen CJ, Halterman WB, et al. Adolescent girls in Maine are at risk for vitamin D insufficiency. J Am Diet Assoc 2005;105:971–4.
6. Kumar J, Muntner P, Kaskel FJ, et al. Prevalence and associations of 25-hydroxyvitamin D deficiency in US children: NHANES 2001-2004. Pediatrics 2009;124:e362–70.
7. Carmeliet G, Dermauw V, Bouillon R. Vitamin D signaling in calcium and bone homeostasis: a delicate balance. Best Pract Res Clin Endocrinol Metab 2015;29(4):621–31.
8. Elder CJ, Bishop NJ. Rickets. Lancet 2014;383(9929):1665–76.
9. St. Arnaud R, Naja RP. Vitamin D metabolism, cartilage and bone fracture repair. Mol Cell Endocrinol 2011;347:48–54.
10. Brinker MR, O'Connor DP, Monla YT, et al. Metabolic and endocrine abnormalities in patients with nonunions. J Orthop Trauma 2007;21(8):557–70.
11. Pourfeizi HH, Tabriz A, Elmi A, et al. Prevalence of vitamin D deficiency and secondary hyperparathyroidism in nonunion of traumatic fractures. Acta Med Iran 2013;51:705–10.
12. Al-Said YA, Al-Rached HS, Al-Qahtani HA, et al. Severe proximal myopathy with remarkable recovery after vitamin D treatment. Can J Neurol Sci 2009;36:336–9.
13. Prineas JW, Mason AS, Henson RA. Myopathy in metabolic bone disease. Br Med J 1965;1:1034–6.
14. Bischoff-Ferrari HA, Dawson-Hughes B, Orav EJ, et al. Monthly high-dose vitamin D treatment for the prevention of functional decline: a randomised clinical trial. JAMA Intern Med 2016;176:175–83.
15. Plotnikoff GA, Quigley JM. Prevalence of severe hypovitaminosis D in patients with persistent, nonspecific musculoskeletal pain. Mayo Clin Proc 2003;78:1463–70. Available at: http://www.sciencedirect.com/science/article/pii/S0025619611627420.

16. Tague SE, Clarke GL, Winter MK, et al. Vitamin D deficiency promotes skeletal muscle hypersensitivity and sensory hyperinnervation. J Neurosci 2011;31. 13728013738.
17. Grant WB. An estimate of the global reduction in mortality rates through doubling vitamin D levels. Eur J Clin Nutr 2011;65(9):1016–26.
18. Binkley N, Ramamurthy R, Krueger D. Low vitamin D status: definition, prevalence, consequences, and correction. Endocrinol Metab Clin North Am 2010; 39:287–301.
19. Dawson-Hughes B, Heaney RP, Holick MR, et al. Estimates of optimal vitamin D status. Osteoporos Int 2005;16:713–6.
20. Holick MF, Chen TC. Vitamin D deficiency: a worldwide problem with health consequences. Am J Clin Nutr 2008;87:1080S–6S.
21. Hagenau T, Vest R, Gissel TN, et al. Global vitamin D levels in relation to age, gender, skin pigmentation and latitude: an ecologic meta-regression analysis. Osteoporos Int 2009;20:133–40.
22. Ginde AA, Liu MC, Camargo CA. Demographic differences and trends of vitamin D insufficiency in the US population, 1988-2004. Arch Intern Med 2009;169: 626–32.
23. Yetley EA. Assessing the vitamin D status of the US population. Am J Clin Nutr 2008;88:558S–64S.
24. DeLuca HF. Overview of general physiologic features and function of vitamin D. Am J Clin Nutr 2004;80(6 suppl):1689S–96S.
25. Amling M, Priemel M, Holzmann T, et al. Rescue of the skeletal phenotype of vitamin D receptor-ablated mice in the setting of normal mineral ion homeostasis: formal histomorphometric and biomechanical analyses. Endocrinology 1999;140: 4982–7.
26. Fischer V, Haffner-Luntzer M, Amling M, et al. Calcium and vitamin D in bone fracture healing and post-traumatic bone turnover. Eur Cell Mater 2018;35:365–85.
27. Jones G. Pharmacokinetics of vitamin D toxicity. Am J Clin Nutr 2008;88: 582S–6S.
28. Norman AW. From vitamin D to hormone D: fundamentals of the vitamin D endocrine system essential for good health. Am J Clin Nutr 2008;88(2):4915–95.
29. Alshahrani F, Aljohani N. Vitamin D deficiency, sufficiency, and toxicity. Nutrients 2013;5:4605–16.
30. Institute of Medicine, Food and Nutrition Board. Dietary reference intakes for calcium and vitamin D. Washington, DC: National Academy Press; 2010.
31. Holick MF, Binkley NC, Bischoff-Ferarri HA, et al. Evaluation, treatment, and prevention of vitamin D deficiency: an Endocrine Society clinical practice guideline. J Clin Endocrinol Metab 2011;96:1911–30.
32. Trang HM, Cole DE, Rubin LA, et al. Evidence that vitamin D_3 increases serum 25-hydroxyvitamin D more efficiently than does vitamin D_2. Am J Clin Nutr 1998;68: 854–8.
33. Romagnoli E, Mascia ML, Cipriani C, et al. Short and long-term variations in serum calciotropic hormones after a single very large dose of ergocalciferol (vitamin D_2) or cholecalciferol (vitamin D_3) in the elderly. J Clin Endocrinol Metab 2008;93:3015–20.
34. Houghton LA, Vieth R. The case against ergocalciferol (vitamin D-2) as a vitamin supplement. Am J Clin Nutr 2006;84:694–7.
35. Tripkovic L, Lambert H, Hart K, et al. Comparison of vitamin D_2 and vitamin D_3 supplementation in raising serum 25-hydroxyvitamin D status: a systematic review and meta-analysis. Am J Clin Nutr 2012;95:1357–64.

36. Burt LA, Billington EO, Rose MS, et al. Effect of high-dose vitamin D supplementation on volumetric bone density and bone strength: a randomized clinical trial. JAMA 2019;322(8):736–45.

37. Bhamb N, Kanim L, Maldonado R, et al. Effect of modulating dietary vitamin D on the general health of rats during posterolateral spinal fusion. J Orthop Res 2018; 36(5):1435–43.

38. Jingushi S, Iwaki A, Higuchi O, et al. Serum 1 alpha,25-dihydroxyvitamin D_3 accumulates into the fracture callus during rat femoral fracture healing. Endocrinology 1998;139(4):1467–73.

39. Lidor C, Atkin I, Omoy A, et al. Healing of rachitic lesions in chicks by 24,25-dihydroxycholecalciferol administered locally into bone. J Bone Miner Res 1987; 2(2):91–8.

40. Meyr AJ, Mirmiran R, Naldo J, et al. American College of Foot and Ankle Surgeons® clinical consensus statement: perioperative management. J Foot Ankle Surg 2017;56:336–56.

41. Sprague S, Petrisor B, Scott T, et al. What is the role of Vitamin D supplementation in acute fracture patients? A systematic review and meta-analysis of the prevalence of hypovitaminosis D and supplementation efficacy. J Orthop Trauma 2016;30(2):53–63.

42. Hood MA, Murtha YM, Della Rocca GJ, et al. Prevalence of low vitamin D levels in patients with orthopaedic trauma. Am J Orthop 2016;45:ES22–6.

43. Steele B, Serota A, Helfet DL, et al. Vitamin D deficiency: a common occurrence in both high- and low-energy fractures. HSS J 2008;4:143–8.

44. Zellner BS, Dawson JR, Reichel LM, et al. Prospective nutritional analysis of a diverse trauma population demonstrates substantial hypovitaminosis D. J Orthop Trauma 2014;28:e210–5.

45. Lee GH, Lim JW, Park YG, et al. Vitamin D deficiency is highly concomitant but not strong risk factor for mortality in patients aged 50 years and older with hip fractures. J Bone Metab 2015;22:205–9.

46. Leboff MS, Kohlmeier L, Hurwitz S, et al. Occult vitamin D deficiency in postmenopausal US women with acute hip fracture. JAMA 1999;281:1505–11.

47. Diamond T, Smerdely P, Kormas N, et al. Hip fracture in elderly men: the importance of subclinical vitamin D deficiency and hypogonadism. Med J Aust 1998; 169:138–41.

48. Smith JT, Halim K, Palms DA, et al. Prevalence of vitamin D deficiency in patients with foot and ankle injuries. Foot Ankle Int 2014;35:8–13.

49. Aujla RS, Allen PE, Ribbans WJ. Vitamin D levels in 577 consecutive elective foot & ankle surgery patients. Foot Ankle Surg 2019;25:310–5.

50. Moore KR, Howell MA, Saltrick KR, et al. Risk factors associated with nonunion after elective foot and ankle reconstruction: a case-control study. J Foot Ankle Surg 2017;56:457–62.

51. Michelson JD, Charlson MD. Vitamin D Status in an elective orthopedic surgical population. Foot Ankle Int 2016;37(2):186–91.

52. Hanley DA, Davison KS. Vitamin D insufficiency in North America. J Nutr 2005; 135:332–7.

53. Nino S, Soin SP, Avilucea FR. Vitamin D and metabolic supplementation in orthopedic trauma. Orthop Clin North Am 2019;50:171–9.

54. DeFontes K, Smith JT. Surgical considerations for vitamin D deficiency in foot and ankle surgery. Orthop Clin North Am 2019;50:259–67.

55. Fentaw Y, Woldie H, Mekonnen S, et al. Change in serum level of vitamin D and associated factors at early phase of bone healing among fractured adult patients at University of Gondor teaching hospital, Northwest Ethiopia: a prospective follow up study. Nutr J 2017;16(54):1–9.
56. Childs BR, Andres BA, Vallier HA. Economic benefit of calcium and vitamin D supplementation: does it outweigh the cost of nonunion? J Orthop Trauma 2016;30:e285–8.

Plantar Verrucae in Human Immunodeficiency Virus Infection

25 Years of Research of a Viral Coinfection

Check for updates

Jean Paul Dardet[a], Nicholas Patrick Blasingame, BS[b],
Daniel Okpare, BS[b], Luke Leffler, BS[b], Peter Barbosa, PhD[c],*

KEYWORDS

- HIV • HPV • Plantar warts • Plantar verrucae • Immunocompromised
- Antiretroviral therapy

KEY POINTS

- Plantar verrucae, caused by human papillomavirus, are observed at higher rates in human immunodeficiency virus-infected patients.
- Atypical types of human papillomavirus have been identified as causative agents of plantar warts in human immunodeficiency virus-infected patients.
- The implementation of human immunodeficiency virus antiretroviral therapy had an impact on the clinical manifestations of plantar warts, but the prevalence continues to be significantly higher among patients with human immunodeficiency virus infection.
- A limited number of studies have explored treatment modalities for plantar warts in human immunodeficiency virus-infected patients.

INTRODUCTION

Human papillomavirus (HPV) is the causative agent of multiple types of warts in humans, including plantar and skin warts.[1] It is a nonenveloped, double-stranded DNA virus of the *Papillomaviridae* family. There have been more than 180 types of HPV identified, and the virus is known to be strictly epitheliotropic.[2] HPV is pervasive in the human population, with a majority of those infected exhibiting no symptoms.[3]

Certain HPV types are correlated with clinical manifestations in specific locations. For example, HPV types 1, 2, and 4 have been associated with plantar warts.[4,5]

[a] Universidad del Sagrado Corazón, PO Box 12383, San Juan, PR 00914-8505, USA; [b] New York College of Podiatric Medicine, 53 East 124th Street, New York, NY 10035, USA; [c] Natural Sciences Department, Universidad del Sagrado Corazón, PO Box 12383, San Juan, PR 00914-8505, USA
* Corresponding author.
E-mail address: peter.barbosa@sagrado.edu

Clin Podiatr Med Surg 37 (2020) 317–325
https://doi.org/10.1016/j.cpm.2019.12.010
0891-8422/20/© 2019 Elsevier Inc. All rights reserved.
podiatric.theclinics.com

Plantar warts, also known as *plantar verruca*, are an infection of the epithelial keratino-cytes by HPV. Most commonly, these warts manifest on areas of the plantar aspect of the foot, which are subject to high mechanical pressure. Breached skin, primarily caused by microtrauma, is the primary portal of entry for HPV. Infection is most likely to occur after the viral particles are exposed to the basal layer of the skin. It is esti-mated that the annual incidence rate of plantar warts is 14%, with as much as 2% of the healthy population requiring medical care.[3] Certain populations, such as those who are immunocompromised, have been found to be at an increased risk for plantar warts, with an estimated 5 times higher rate clinical presentation.[6]

Perhaps the most clinically significant source of immunodeficiency in conjunction with plantar warts is the acquired immunodeficiency syndrome (AIDS) in human immu-nodeficiency virus (HIV) infection. Plantar warts represent one of the main podiatric clinical complications of HIV infection.[6] As of 2018, 37.9 million people are living with HIV worldwide, of which 23.3 million (20.5 million–24.3 million) are receiving highly active antiretroviral therapy (ART) to combat the virus.[7] In the United States, in 2017 it was estimated that 38,600 people above 13 years of age were living with HIV.[8]

With the implementation of highly active ART as a treatment for HIV infection in 1997, the mortality rate for AIDS markedly decreased. The treatment combines 3 or more anti-retroviral pharmacologic agents to reduce viral load and elevate $CD4^+$ T-cell counts in the patient. The increased life expectancy in HIV infection as a result of ART resulted in changes in the podiatric clinical practice in this cohort. In this review, we summarize plantar warts and its clinical correlation during HIV infection. We focus on virologic and epidemiologic aspects of plantar verrucae in HIV infection, and we highlight changes brought about by the implementation of ART. Our review is organized and sources a collection of case reports, small trials, and epidemiologic studies over the past 25 years.

METHODS

We have performed a systematic review of literature concerning the clinical manifes-tations of plantar verrucae in HIV-infected patients. The specifications in search criteria for articles published with open start date until June 2019. Two search engines were used for selection of publications: PubMed and Google Scholar. The following terms related to plantar warts were used in the database exploration: plantar verrucae, plantar warts, HPV, and human papillomavirus. The following terms related to HIV infection were used in the database exploration: HIV, AIDS, and human immunodefi-ciency virus. Searches were conducted with all possible combinations including one of the terms in each of the 2 categories (plantar warts and HIV). We identified 47 related reports in the combined search of PubMed Database and Google Scholar. Exclusion criteria included articles not written in English, or articles that did not include both categories. Inclusion criteria included articles that covered both primary topics in the same report, plantar warts and HIV. Amid these criteria, 25 articles concerning plantar verrucae in HIV-infected patients were included.

CASE REPORTS

Case reports of HIV-infected patients with concurrent HPV infection manifested as warts can be divided into 3 primary categories. Reports published in the 1990s illus-trated the connection between the clinical manifestation of warts in this population. They served to incite the possibility that plantar warts demonstrated a different clinical profile in HIV-infected patients. Case reports in the early 2000s shed light onto the impact of treatment, either specific against the wart or as a consequence of HIV ART. The more recent case reports focused viral typing of atypical HPV species.

The manifestation of highly resistant plantar verrucae in HIV infection is demonstrated pre-ART implementation by Soltani and colleagues[9] (1996) case study report. A 26-year-old man with multiple bilateral, large hyperkeratotic lesions presented in 1992 to the Pacific Coast Hospital in San Francisco. The verrucae lesions were found on both feet under the hallux, first, second, and fourth metatarsal heads, and third and fourth interspaces. Medical history indicated the patient had tested positive for HIV 3 years prior, although the patient had a CD4$^+$ count of 525 cells/mm^3 2 years after starting treatment for plantar verrucae, suggestive of a noncompromised immune system. After 5 years of treatment, the plantar verrucae showed full recurrence despite treatment with debridement, liquid nitrogen, salicylic acid, topical 5-fluorouracil, and enucleation by blunt dissection.[9] The patient, being relatively immunocompetent, was an early suggestion that viral interactions between HPV and HIV may influence highly recurrent, aggressive plantar verrucae.

Two related case reports were presented in 1999 and 2002, which provided an indication that improved immune function could alter the course of warts. The first report detailed the case of a 28-year-old man who acquired HIV in the early 1980s and presented with a worsening hand verruca in 1988. The patient had no improvement despite therapy for the warts, until a protease-inhibitor was added to the patient's ART in October 1996. In early 1997, the appearance of the hand verrucae had disappeared, and the 1-year checkup, the warts remained absent. No therapy against HPV that would have affected the warts was started when ART with a protease inhibitor was implemented.[10] Another case study that supports regression of verrucae owing to the implementation of ART was done on a 34-year-old patient with HIV with aggressive verrucae. Four months after the patient started a strictly monitored ART treatment program, total regression of the verrucae was observed.[11] Although both of these studies involved hand warts and not plantar lesions, they have shown ART adherence is beneficial to surmounting HPV in the presence of HIV owing to an increase in cellular immunity.

Two case studies have identified unusual HPV types present in lesions of HIV-positive individuals, including HPV-66 and HPV-69.[12,13] A 37-year-old HIV-positive patient presented with a large verrucous plaque on the right heel that extended up the patient's medial and lateral aspects of the foot. Differential diagnosis included bacterial/fungal infection, squamous cell carcinoma, and verrucous carcinoma. A biopsy showed viral changes, papillomatosis, acanthosis, hyperkeratosis, and superficial telangiectasia. Polymerase chain reaction confirmed HPV infection by identifying HPV types 11, 16, 53, and 66 in the patient's foot plaque. HPV-66 is typically associated with the HPV infections of the cervix and is extremely uncommon in plantar verrucae. Identifying a common cervical HPV type in plantar verrucae led to a gynecologic examination in this patient detecting cervical dysplasia owing to HPV types 11, 16, 52, 53, and 66.[12] In a separate case study report, another rare type HPV was confirmed in a HIV-positive patient with a clinically aggressive lesion. The 57-year-old man presented with a circular 18-mm diameter lesion under his first metatarsal head. A biopsy, followed by DNA extraction and amplification, led to the first detection of HPV-69 in plantar verrucae.[13]

HUMAN PAPILLOMA VIRUS VIRAL TYPING

Although HPV-1, -2, and -4 have been linked to the development of plantar verrucae in classic literature,[4,5,14] more recent studies highlight increased incidence of HPV-27 and -57 in cutaneous lesions, including plantar surfaces.[15–17] The virologic question of HPV typing in plantar verrucae lesions from HIV-infected patients has been the research subject of a number of publications. As described, 2 case reports have identified atypical HPV types 66 and 69 in plantar lesions from HIV-infected patients.[12,13] In addition to these single-patient reports, larger trials have analyzed HPV viral typing in HIV-infected cohorts.

In a prospective study in Brazil by Porro and colleagues[18] (2003), 25 samples of common warts from 24 patients infected with HIV and from 13 control individuals with no HIV infection were collected between March 1998 and August 1999. The objective of this study was to determine HPV types found in cutaneous warts of HIV-infected patients and to compare the results with those in immunocompetent patients. Twenty-four HIV-infected patients (14 men and 10 women; age range, 21–44 years) were included in this study. The duration of warts among HIV-infected patients varied from 6 months to 10 years. Five different HPV types were found in the HIV-infected cohort, and only 1 HPV type was detected in each lesion. The most frequent HPV type was HPV-2, identified in 38% of the samples. HPV-57 was found in 31%, HPV-27 and HPV-6 were each detected in 12%, and HPV-7 was identified in 6% of the samples. HPV types 2, 27, and 57 prevailed in both groups, HIV-infected and noninfected cohorts. However, HPV-6, s genital type rarely found in cutaneous lesions, was detected in 2 warts from HIV-infected patients and in 1 lesion of the immunocompetent group. HPV-7, more commonly linked to butcher's warts, was found in a nonfacial lesion of an HIV-infected patient.[18] It must be clarified that this study included a variety of common warts, most of which were not plantar lesions.

King and colleagues[19] (2014) examined 39 lesions from 17 individuals, exclusively plantar warts. Their study also compared HIV-infected and noninfected patients; 9 HIV-infected, 8 noninfected. Although atypical HPV types were not found in either group, a large proportion of the samples from noninfected individuals typed as HPV-27 (87.5%). HPV-2 was the predominant type identified in HIV-infected individuals (50%). Their study also correlated specific HPV types with the clinical classifications of verruca plantaris, mosaic warts or punctate verrucae.[19]

A summary of atypical HPV types found in plantar verrucae of HIV-infected patients is summarized in **Table 1**.

SMALL TRIALS

This section on small trials covers clinical characterization studies, excluding those related to treatment options or HPV typing previously described. To procure a better understanding of the characteristics of plantar verrucae in HIV patients before the implementation of ART, a study was conducted in 1995 to attempt to answer this question. The objective of study focused on 3 clinical characteristics—the size, number, and clinical type—of plantar verrucae present in HIV-infected and noninfected

Table 1	
Atypical HPV types found in plantar lesions of HIV-infected patients	
Atypical HPV	**Reference**
HPV-6	Porro et al,[18] 2003
HPV-7	Porro et al,[18] 2003
HPV-66	Davis et al,[12] 2000
HPV-66	Whitaker et al,[13] 2001

Data from Refs.[12,13,18]

populations. The findings of this small trial demonstrated that when compared with HIV-negative patients, plantar warts were more numerous and of larger size in the HIV-infected cohort. The study also found that mosaic-type warts were more common in the HIV-infected group.[20]

An analogous small trial was conducted in 2008, more than a decade after the widespread implementation of ART. The findings of this study were in great contrast to those observed in 1995 (before ART implementation). First, when comparing HIV-infected and noninfected individuals in 2008, there were no significant differences in size or number of plantar warts. Moreover, when comparing only the HIV-infected groups from 1995 versus 2008, changes in size and number were noticeable. For wart size, a 47% mean decrease in 2008 was observed, which was nonsignificant ($P = .06$). For number of warts, a 66% mean decrease in the mean per HIV-positive individual was observed, which was significant ($P = .004$).[21]

EPIDEMIOLOGIC STUDIES

Two large-scale studies examined the prevalence of plantar warts among HIV-infected individuals.[6,22] Both of these studies took place in San Francisco, California, and were conducted under similar methodologies. Researchers set up a station at a local street fair, invited participants to complete an anonymous survey including questions on demographics, HIV status, and presence of plantar verrucae lesions. Participants who indicated the presence of plantar warts were invited to have a podiatric clinical examination on site. The key difference between these 2 studies was its tactical timing: in the first study, data were collected in 1995, before the implementation of ART in 1997, and in the second study data were collected in 2008, more than a decade after ART implementation. This strategic design allowed for observing and contrasting prevalence before and after ART, which provided a surrogate analysis of the clinical impact of ART in the manifestation of plantar warts in HIV-positive patients. **Table 2** summarizes and contrasts findings of these studies.

In summary, according to the study conducted in 1995, before the implementation of ART, HIV-positive patients were 10.0 times more likely to develop plantar verrucae. The second study conducted after ART implementation indicated that HIV-positive patients were 5.2 times more likely to develop plantar verrucae than those without HIV infection.[2] This decrease in symptom exacerbation since the implementation of ART was not shown to be statistically significant ($P = .33$).

Table 2
Comparing plantar verrucae rates by HIV status, adjusting for time

HIV status	Prevalence		
	2008	1995	Overall
HIV (+)	20.6%	17.0%	19.1%
HIV (−)	4.8%	2.0%	3.5%
OR (95% CI)	5.2 (2.5–11.0)	10.0 (3.4–29.0)	6.4 (3.5–11.8)
P value	<.0001	<.0001	.33[a]

Abbreviations: CI, confidence interval; OR, odds ratio.
[a] Significant at the .05 level. Overall P value using Breslow-Day test of homogeneity of odds ratios.
Data from Johnston J, King CM, Shanks S, et al. Prevalence of plantar verrucae in patients with human immunodeficiency virus infection during the post-highly active antiretroviral therapy era. Journal of the American Podiatry Association. 2011;101(1):35-40.

Another large-scale study shed some light on the dermatologic complications of HIV infection, including plantar verrucae. This retrospective study had a longitudinal observational design, including a cohort of 965 HIV-positive patients. A total of 333 of these consulted a dermatologist and were included in the final analysis. HPV complications were the most common skin manifestation. Common warts, which included plantar warts, were the third most common clinical manifestation observed in this cohort.[23]

CD4 COUNTS

One of the most reliable clinical indicators of HIV disease progression is the patient's CD4 counts, which represent the number of T-helper cells present in the patient's blood. Because HIV targets T-helper cells, the CD4 count is a surrogate indicator of immune competency in the patient. As CD4 counts fall below normal levels (500–1500 cells/mm³), the patient is considered to be immunocompromised. Based on these parameters, there was an expectation of a correlation between CD4 counts and the extent of severity or counts of plantar warts in this cohort. However, in 3 separate studies where this question was addressed, this expected correlation was not observed. Meberg and colleagues[20] (1998) did not see any correlation between number, size, or clinical type of verrucae and CD4 counts in their HIV-positive cohort. In agreement with other post-ART HPV literature, Nuno-Gonzalez and colleagues[23] (2017) found no correlation between CD4 levels and prevalence of warts. Furthermore, in a post-ART retrospective study out of San Francisco General Hospital's HIV-Dermatology clinic, Mirmirani and colleagues[24] (2002) looked at verrucae among other skin diagnoses to create a Skin Quality of Life Score. A higher Skin Quality of Life Score indicates better skin quality. The study found no correlation between a raised Skin Quality of Life Score and CD4 counts.[24]

TREATMENT

Treatments for plantar warts in the general population are diverse, and range from conservative options to surgical interventions.[3,25] Studies relating to plantar wart treatment specifically in the HIV-positive population are limited. These include 2 case reports, one expert opinion, and one small trial.[10,12,13,26] In **Table 3**, we summarize the treatment modality, type of study and clinical outcome observed in each of these 4 reports. This limited number of studies were all reported from 1999 to 2001.

Table 3
Treatment reports of plantar warts in HIV-positive patients

Treatment Modality	Type of Study	Clinical Outcome	Reference
Immunomodulatory therapy: imiquimod (Aldara)	Expert opinion, clinical review	Full resolution	Conant,[26] 2000
HIV ART	Case report	Full resolution	Spach & Colven,[10] 1999
Topical cidofovir	Case report	Full resolution	Davis et al,[12] 2000
Surgical curettage vs salicylic acid vs control group (no treatment)	Small trial: 37 patients in 3 treatment arms	Recurrence in both treated groups	Whitaker et al,[13] 2001

Data from Refs.[10–13,26]

SUMMARY

This literature review intends to illustrate the onset of clinical manifestations of plantar verrucae in HIV infected patients and to evaluate the impact of the implementation of highly active ART in this population. Plantar verrucae, or simply plantar warts, are common, yet pervasive cutaneous lesions caused by HPV. Although other HPV-infected populations are often asymptomatic, immunocompromised patients have been observed to present an increased number of plantar wart manifestations.[27] Additionally, plantar verrucae in HIV-positive individuals are more clinically aggressive than those found in HIV-negative individuals. According to a post-ART study of the characterization of plantar verrucae among HIV individuals conducted in 1995, patients with HIV infection were 10.0 times more likely to present plantar warts compared with patients who did not present the infection. Furthermore, the results of this study report that the number and size of verrucae were found to be significantly larger in HIV-infected individuals than in their noninfected counterparts.[20,22]

Since the development of antiretroviral therapies, a similar study regarding the prevalence of plantar verrucae in HIV-positive versus HIV-negative individuals (after ART) was conducted in 2008. Comparing the number and size of verrucae lesions between these populations, no statistically significant differences were observed. However, a significant reduction in the number of warts per HIV-infected individual is distinguished from 1995 to the data collected in 2008 ($P = .004$). Evidently, patients with HIV infection in 2008 were still significantly more likely to present plantar verrucae. Analysis of the data demonstrates that patients with HIV infection were 5.2 times more likely to present with plantar verrucae compared to patients without HIV infection in 2008. Hitherto the statistical value of 10.0 reported in 1995, the decrease in prevalence of plantar verrucae among HIV-infected individuals in 2008 is not statistically significantly different ($P = .33$). This evidence is a clear indication that the outbreak of HIV-related podiatric clinical manifestations, such as plantar verrucae, is a prevailing issue in the symptomatic treatment of immunocompromised patients.[6]

Currently, it is estimated that 1.1 million Americans are living with AIDS/HIV and that approximately 38,700 new cases are diagnosed each year.[8] After the implementation of highly active ART and its consequential increase in the life expectancy of patients with HIV infection, it is likely that this patient population will become of greater significance to the field of podiatric medicine. Given that immunocompromised patients are likely to present common podiatric medical issues such as plantar verrucae, prevalence and typing studies could provide a fundamental basis for the treatment modalities in this area of clinical podiatry. The small number of reports relating to treatment modalities offers an opportunity in the podiatric field to investigate in clinical trials what are the most effective plantar wart treatments in HIV-infected patients.

ACKNOWLEDGMENTS

The authors of this article would like to thank Ms Erica B. Benoit for her contributions to the editing of the article.

DISCLOSURE

The authors have nothing to disclose.

REFERENCES

1. Carroll KC, Butel J, Morse S. Jawetz Melnick & Adelbergs medical microbiology 27 E. New York: McGraw Hill Professional; 2015.

2. Colegio OR. Skin diseases in the immunosuppressed. 1st edition. Cham (Switzerland): Springer International Publishing; 2018. https://doi.org/10.1007/978-3-319-68790-2. Available at: https://ebookcentral.proquest.com/lib/[SITE_ID]/detail.action?docID=5439435.

3. Witchey DJ, Witchey NB, Roth-Kauffman MM, et al. Plantar warts: epidemiology, pathophysiology, and clinical management. J Am Osteopath Assoc 2018;118(2): 92–105.

4. Fields BN, Knipe DM, Howley PM. Fields virology. Philadelphia: Wolters Kluwer Health/Lippincott Williams & Wilkins; 2007.

5. Bunney MH, Benton C, Cubie HA. Viral warts: biology and treatment. Oxford (England): Oxford University Press; 1992.

6. Johnston J, King CM, Shanks S, et al. Prevalence of plantar verrucae in patients with human immunodeficiency virus infection during the post-highly active antiretroviral therapy era. J Am Podiatry Assoc 2011;101(1):35–40. Available at: https://www.ncbi.nlm.nih.gov/pubmed/21242468.

7. AIDSinfo UNAIDS. 2019. Available at: http://aidsinfo.unaids.org. Accessed August 23, 2019.

8. CDC HIV basics. 2019. Available at: https://www.cdc.gov/hiv/basics/statistics. html. Accessed July 27, 2017.

9. Soltani SK, Kenyon E, Barbosa P. Chronic and aggressive plantar verrucae in a patient with HIV. J Am Podiatr Med Assoc 1996;86(11):555–8. Available at: https://www.ncbi.nlm.nih.gov/pubmed/8961659.

10. Spach DH, Colven R. Resolution of recalcitrant hand warts in an HIV-infected patient treated with potent antiretroviral therapy. J Am Acad Dermatol 1999;40(5): 818–21. Available at: https://www.sciencedirect.com/science/article/pii/S0190962299000109.

11. Turnbull JR, Husak R, Treudler R, et al. Regression of multiple viral warts in a human immunodeficiency virus-infected patient treated by triple antiretroviral therapy. Br J Dermatol 2002;146(2):330. Available at: https://onlinelibrary.wiley.com/doi/abs/10.1046/j.0007-0963.2001.04660.x.

12. Davis MDP, Gostout BS, Persing DH, et al. Large plantar wart caused by human papillomavirus-66 and resolution by topical cidofovir therapy. J Am Acad Dermatol 2000;43(2):340–3. Available at: https://www.sciencedirect.com/science/article/pii/S0190962200702878.

13. Whitaker JM, Gaggero GL, Loveland L, et al. Plantar verrucae in patients with human immunodeficiency virus. clinical presentation and treatment response. J Am Podiatr Med Assoc 2001;91(2):79–84.

14. Green M, Orth G, Wold WS, et al. Analysis of human cancers, normal tissues, and verruce plantares for DNA sequences of human papillomavirus types 1 and 2. Virology 1981;110(1):176–84.

15. Chan S, Chew S, Egawa K, et al. Phylogenetic analysis of the human papillomavirus type 2 (HPV-2), HPV-27, and HPV-57 group, which is associated with common warts. Virology 1997;239(2):296–302. Available at: http://www.sciencedirect.com/science/article/pii/S0042682297988966.

16. Rubben A, Kalka K, Spelten B, et al. Clinical features and age distribution of patients with HPV 2/27/57-induced common warts. Arch Dermatol Res 1997;289(6): 337–40.

17. Tomson N, Sterling J, Ahmed I, et al. Human papillomavirus typing of warts and response to cryotherapy. J Eur Acad Dermatol Venereol 2011;25(9):1108–11. Available at: https://onlinelibrary.wiley.com/doi/abs/10.1111/j.1468-3083.2010.03906.x.

18. Porro AM, Alchorne MMA, Mota GR, et al. Detection and typing of human papillomavirus in cutaneous warts of patients infected with human immunodeficiency virus type 1. Br J Dermatol 2003;149(6):1192–9. Available at: http://www.ingentaconnect.com/content/bsc/bjd/2003/00000149/00000006/art00011.
19. King CM, Johnston JS, Ofili K, et al. Human papillomavirus types 2, 27, and 57 identified in plantar verrucae from HIV-positive and HIV-negative subjects. J Am Podiatr Med Assoc 2014;104(2):141–6.
20. Meberg R, Kenyon E, Bierman R, et al. Characterization of plantar verrucae among individuals with human immunodeficiency virus. J Am Podiatr Med Assoc 1998;88(9):442–5. Available at: http://www.ncbi.nlm.nih.gov/pubmed/9770936.
21. Afesllari E, Miller TJ, Huchital MJ, et al. Reduction in size and number of plantar verrucae in human immunodeficiency virus–infected individuals after the implementation of highly active antiretroviral therapy. J Am Podiatr Med Assoc 2015; 105(5):401–6.
22. Kenyon E, Loveland L, Kilpatrick R, et al. Epidemiology of plantar verrucae in HIV-infected individuals. J Acquir Immune Defic Syndr Hum Retrovirol 1998; 17(1):94–5.
23. Nuno-Gonzalez A, Losa Garcia JE, López Estebaranz JL, et al. Human papilloma virus dermatosis in human immunodeficiency virus-positive patients: a 14-year retrospective study in 965 patients. Med Clin (Barc) 2017;148(9):401–4. Available at: https://www.sciencedirect.com/science/article/pii/S2387020617302772.
24. Mirmirani P, Maurer TA, Berger TG, et al. Skin-related quality of life in HIV-infected patients on highly active antiretroviral therapy. J Cutan Med Surg 2002;6(1):10–5. Available at: https://journals.sagepub.com/doi/full/10.1177/120347540200600102.
25. Vlahovic TC, Khan MT. The human papillomavirus and its role in plantar warts: a comprehensive review of diagnosis and management. Clin Podiatr Med Surg 2016;33(3):337–53.
26. Conant MA. Immunomodulatory therapy in the management of viral infections in patients with HIV infection. J Am Acad Dermatol 2000;43(1):S30.
27. Ghadgepatil SS, Gupta S, Sharma YK. Clinicoepidemiological study of different types of warts. Dermatol Res Pract 2016;2016:7989817.

VII. Dr. William M. Scholl College of Podiatric Medicine

The Role of the Podiatrist in Assessing and Reducing Fall Risk: An Updated Review

Noah J. Rosenblatt, PhD*, Christopher Girgis, DPM,
Marco Avalos, MD, Adam E. Fleischer, DPM, Ryan T. Crews, MS

KEYWORDS

- Balance • Older adults • Surgery • Shoe modification • Prevention • Pain • Falls

KEY POINTS

- The process of preventing falls should commence by taking an in-depth medical history during initial interaction with a patient.
- When conducting a lower extremity physical examination with an emphasis on fall prevention, it is important to consider foot biomechanics, foot problems and deformities, and footwear.
- Multifactorial interventions that include a combination of podiatric care, footwear assessment, and distribution of prefabricated insoles with exercises seem effective at reducing falls.
- Insole features including thickness, texture, and softness could impact effectiveness with regard to fall prevention.
- General foot and podiatric care to address pain and problems (eg, debriding hyperkeratosis, nail care) may improve strength, balance, and function.

INTRODUCTION

With approximately one out of every three persons aged greater than or equal to 65 years falling each year,[1] falls present a tremendous challenge to health care systems. Recent estimates indicate that by 2030 older adults will incur 11.9 million fall injuries per year in the United States alone "unless effective interventions are implemented nationwide."[1] As part of the Centers for Disease Control and Prevention's Stopping Elderly Accidents, Deaths & Injuries Initiative, an algorithm has been created to assist health care providers in fall risk screening, assessment, and intervention.[2] That algorithm specifically recommends referring patients to podiatrists when feet/footwear issues are identified. However, podiatrists are content experts in several

Dr. William M. Scholl College of Podiatric Medicine's Center for Lower Extremity Ambulatory Research (CLEAR), 3333 Green Bay Road, North Chicago, IL 60064, USA
* Corresponding author.
E-mail address: noah.rosenblatt@rosalindfranklin.edu

Clin Podiatr Med Surg 37 (2020) 327–369
https://doi.org/10.1016/j.cpm.2019.12.005
0891-8422/20/© 2019 Elsevier Inc. All rights reserved.

of the modifiable risk factors to be assessed as part of the algorithm (eg, evaluating gait and balance, and assessing feet/footwear), and therefore have an important role to play in identifying and mitigating fall risk. In recognition of podiatry's potential to help combat falls by older adults, in 2013 the *Journal of the American Podiatric Medical Association* devoted a special issue to falls prevention.[3] In addition to seven original research studies, that special issue included a systematic review regarding footwear interventions and balance[4] and a systematic review and meta-analysis on the use of foot and ankle (FA) exercise for reducing fall risk.[5] Here we present an updated review of the literature, with the goal of providing new insight on the topic and a broader review of podiatry's role to play in the prevention of falls. Our choice to write this review was also driven by our specific research interests at the Dr. William M. Scholl College of Podiatric Medicine focused on the prevention of falls by older adults and at-risk populations.[6–20]

METHODS: SEARCH CRITERIA AND INCLUDED STUDIES

A search of the PubMed electronic database was completed from April 8–12, 2019 using the following original search inquiries for studies completed in the last 5 years: "balanc* AND amputat*," "balanc* AND podiatr* treatment" and "balanc* AND podiatr*," "balanc* AND amput*," "podiatr* surgery AND balance," "foot surgery AND balance." After removing duplicates, a single fourth year podiatry student (C.G.) screened articles for inclusion. Article titles were initially used to screen for irrelevant publications, during which time most of the initial search returns were excluded. For example, such titles as "Isolated Fracture of the Medial Cuneiform" or "Effectiveness of the Bobath Concept in the Treatment of Stroke: A Systematic Review" were deemed irrelevant to podiatric involvement in fall prevention. The abstracts for articles with pertinent titles were screened to make final determinations of inclusion in this review. A total of 41 articles were deemed appropriate for inclusion.

The full text of all included articles was read by the same podiatric medical student and the following information was extracted (**Tables 1** and **2**): study design, patient population, pertinent methods including assessment tools and/or interventions used, study setting, and main conclusions/results. In addition, for each article the Oxford Center for Evidence-based Medicine resource was used to provide the level of evidence for the study. We then separated articles into two categories: articles related to fall risk assessment and articles related to interventions to reduce fall risk. Importantly, a study did not need to include falls as a primary outcome to be included in this review. Studies with outcomes that included measures of balance or gait were also considered.

Although the current review emphasizes recent work in the area of podiatry and falls, additional relevant articles are included based on references within the included studies and the authors' knowledge of the relevant literature.

RESULTS: IDENTIFYING FALL RISK
Assessing Risk Factors Through Podiatric and Medical History

The process of preventing falls should commence by taking an in-depth medical history during initial interaction with a patient. Although most podiatric histories enquire about foot pain, doing so is particularly important when assessing fall risk. According to Dunn and colleagues,[21] foot pain affects approximately one-third of community-dwelling people older than the age of 65, and a clinical evaluation of 417 people aged 61 years and older living in residential care facilities found that 84% of residents had at least one foot complaint, the most common of which was

Table 1
Summary of recent studies related to fall-risk assessment

Citation	Study Design (Level of Evidence)	Patients	Pertinent Methods	Setting	How Risk (Effects) Assessed?	Conclusion/Findings
Risk assessment via general medical history (diseases, medications, prior amputation)						
Morpeth et al,[31] 2016	Case-control (level 3)	42 women (21 with RA, 21 control subjects)	Foot disability and impairment were measured using LFIS, walking velocity measured using GAITRite, FoF using FES-I	Outpatient	Correlations (foot problems and FoF); group comparison (FoF and foot problems in RA vs control)	In people with RA, foot impairment and disability (from LFIS) are significantly correlated with FoF (a risk factor for falling); RA had significantly greater FoF and foot disability and impairment
Kunkel et al,[34] 2017	Cross-sectional observational (level 3)	23 stroke patients 23 control subjects	Participants completed tests assessing sensation, FPI, FFI, ankle dorsiflexion and first MPJ ROM, HV presence and severity, fall history	Home visits	Between-group differences (stroke vs control and stroke fallers vs nonfallers)	Differences between the affected side and nonaffected side were seen in sensation and ROM of the first MPJ; compared with the control group, stroke patients had reduced sensation, higher FPI and FFI scores; pooled FPI data showed stroke fallers have significantly greater foot pronation than nonfallers

(continued on next page)

Table 1
(continued)

Citation	Study Design (Level of Evidence)	Patients	Pertinent Methods	Setting	How Risk (Effects) Assessed?	Conclusion/Findings
Cherry et al,[33] 2017	Cross-sectional (level 3)	182 SLE patients	Survey about: lower limb circulation health, lower limb nerve function, foot and ankle skin health, lower limb musculoskeletal health, receive or needed foot and ankle treatments	Survey	Falls history seems to have been reported in the nerve function section; description of prevalence of foot problems in SLE population	16% reported sensory neuropathy and 25% reported a fall caused by altered sensation; 85% reported some form of circulatory impairment; 86% reported some form of foot and ankle skin health complaint (most frequent was calluses or corn formation); 87% reported some form of musculoskeletal complication (most joint pain)

				Fall history at the completion of the study	Fall odds were significantly heightened for participants with vascular comorbidities (OR, 3.46), although vascular (vs traumatic) amputation was associated with reduced odds (OR, .038); TFA was also associated with reduced risk relative to TTA (OR, 0.08; 95% CI, 0.01–0.82); although age was not significant there was an age × level interaction with older TFA having higher risk (age × TFA, OR, 1.06); having better balance increased fall odds (OR, 23.29), but there was a balance × confidence interaction where high confidence and high balance reduced the odds of falls (OR, 0.27)
Wong & Chihuri,[35] 2019	Cross-sectional study (level 3)	305 community PLL (138 TTA and 105 TFA)	Retrospective analysis of baseline data from PLL participating in a large prospective longitudinal cohort study; participant self-reported balance confidence, prosthetics function; gait and balance assessed with BBS, TUG and 2-min-walk test; fall history from records	Clinic	

(continued on next page)

Table 1
(continued)

Citation	Study Design (Level of Evidence)	Patients	Pertinent Methods	Setting	How Risk (Effects) Assessed?	Conclusion/Findings
Aprile et al,[37] 2018	Case-control (level 4)	18 participants (6 diabetic with first ray amputation, 6 diabetic without amputation, and 6 healthy)	Gait analysis performed with a 3-dimensional motion capture system; QoL and pain self-reported	Gait laboratory	Between-group comparisons	The amputee group walked significantly slower than and had wider and longer steps than and had greater peak hip flexion than the 2 other groups; amputation impacts kinematic parameters of walking are different than the other 2 groups; pain was higher and more often in the ADP group
Hunter et al,[36] 2019	Prospective cohort study (level 2)	27 unilateral lower extremity amputees (TTA, TFA), >50 y old	Provided surveys regarding falls and balance confidence during rehabilitation and 4 mo after discharge		Report of falls during rehabilitation and during 4 mo after (recall of events at the end of the program and 4 mo after)	While in rehabilitation 2 participants reported falling and 2 said fear of falling affected activity; at 4 mo 8 reported falling with only 2 wearing the prosthesis and 7 said fear of falling interfered with ADLs; balance confidence did not significantly improve at 4 mo

Kerkhoff et al,[77] 2018	Case series (level 4)	8 patients with ankle fusion patients	Participants walked at self-pace, and fast and PS was assessed with and without vision on a rigid surface and foam	Gait laboratory	Comparison of spatiotemporal gait parameters and balance between limbs	Fused ankle showed a decreased contact time, reduced ROM while walking; greater knee ROM on fused ankle side while walking; COP velocity on foam was significantly higher on contralateral limb compared with fused limb; unaffected leg may compensate for affected leg for balance
Risk assessment via podiatric history (eg, foot deformities, LLD)						
Pratelli et al,[87] 2017	Case series (level 4)	52 Patients with clinical heterometry >5 mm	Examination of LLD with balance board (Body Lizard 3.0 (Body barycenter and weight imbalance); effect of wedge under the hypometric limb heel on weight imbalance evaluated	Postural clinic	Association between LLD and weight imbalance	Most patients with clinical heterometry show a weight imbalance on the longer limb; only 21/52 patients showed an improvement in weight imbalance in the wedge position; correction of LLD may not result in positive outcomes for all and benefits of correction in terms of stability (weight balance) should be checked after made

(continued on next page)

Table 1
(continued)

Citation	Study Design (Level of Evidence)	Patients	Pertinent Methods	Setting	How Risk (Effects) Assessed?	Conclusion/Findings
Muchna et al,[24] 2018	Retrospective cohort study (level 3)	117 older adults (90 with foot problems, 27 without foot problems)	Foot problems (yes) if: self-reported pain, or visually identified deformity (eg, bunion, hammertoe, flatfoot), or VPT >25 or nonresponsive to monofilament on first metatarsal head or heel; frailty if >2/5 on a 5-point assessment; fall history (6 mo prior) and prospective falls over 6 mo after recruitment; gait and balance, physical activities	In-home assessments	Fall history (6 mo recall) and prospective falls (6 mo after, through a fall diary log)	Foot problems were not significantly associated with falls in the 6 mo before or following inclusion in the study; presence of foot problems (pain, peripheral neuropathy, or deformity) increased with frailty (OR, 8.3 for frail vs nonfrail); foot pain and neuropathy were associated with changes in gait and balance (eg, increased postural sway) and physical activity; concern about falls was higher in those with foot problems
Koura et al,[47] 2017	Cross-sectional (level 3)	40 (20 bilateral flat feet, 20 normal feet)	Dynamic balance (Biodex balance system) based on 3 stability indices	Gait laboratory	Between-group comparison of stability	The group with flat feet showed significantly impaired stability for all 3 measures when under level 4 difficulty (on an 8-level scale with level 8 being the most stabilizing) but no differences at level 8

Bowen et al,[32] 2016	Retrospective cohort study (level 3)	218 Parkinson and 145 poststroke patients	Survey of footwear characteristic, frequency of foot problems, and fall history	In home	Retrospective falls (12-mo recall)	A significantly greater proportion of fallers reported foot problems (57% vs 41%) and a significantly greater proportion of fallers reported that foot problems influenced their balance (34% vs 21%); factors affecting choice of footwear are discussed
Saghazadeh et al,[48] 2015	Cross-sectional (level 3)	140 community-dwelling older women	2 PS measures taken by force plate; sitting and standing navicular height and foot mobility; 3 groups defined for each of sitting and standing: low, medium, and high arch; 3 groups for mobility: low, medium, or high navicular drop	Health center	Analysis of covariances to compare PS between foot groups after accounting for age, body mass index, and diseases	Significant effect of group (based on sitting arch height) for both PS measures with post hoc indicating worse PS in low vs high arch for 1 measure; no significant effect of group (based on standing arch height) on either PS measure; significant effect of group (based on foot mobility) for one PS measure with no significant post hoc tests; sitting navicular height and foot mobility are associated with postural sway in elderly women

(continued on next page)

Table 1
(continued)

Citation	Study Design (Level of Evidence)	Patients	Pertinent Methods	Setting	How Risk (Effects) Assessed?	Conclusion/Findings
Chen et al,[46] 2014	Prospective cohort study (level 2)	26 patients with chronic ankle instability (11 functional; 15 mechanical), 14 healthy control subjects	Single limb PS test performed 3 times with and without vision; sway reported in 4 directions	Gait laboratory	Comparison of PS between groups with post hoc test	With vision, the group with mechanical instability presented increased sway (relative to control) in 1 direction on affected limb and separate direction on unaffected limb; without vision the mechanical instability group presented increased sway in 3 directions on the affected side and 1 direction on the unaffected side; no differences were found for any measure of PS for patients with functional instability compared with control subjects

Risk assessment via footwear

Donovan-Hall et al,[51] 2019	Case series (level 4)	15 stroke patients (8 men, 7 women)	Semistructured interviews to determine impact of stroke and foot problems; footwear choice and priorities; issues and challenges with footwear	Survey in home	Effect of stroke over mobility and foot care changes	11/15 had impaired mobility, being weakness and loss of sensation the main factors to affect gait; endurance problems were associated with unsteadiness; one-third of patients experienced numbness or altered sensation; other foot problems noted include foot drop, burning cramps, and fluid retention; foot changes caused by edema have created an inconvenience to find appropriate shoes

(continued on next page)

Table 1
(continued)

Citation	Study Design (Level of Evidence)	Patients	Pertinent Methods	Setting	How Risk (Effects) Assessed?	Conclusion/Findings
Other						
Dixon et al,[88] 2017	Systematic review of balance measured used for patient with diabetes and DPN (level 1)	8 articles that included patients with diabetes (6 with DPN)	10 different balance measures were identified in the 8 included studies		Effects of type 2 diabetes mellitus and DPN on balance	TUG was most commonly used (in 4 of 8 studies); BBS, TUG, FRT, Tinetti Performance Oriented Mobility Assessment, and Tandem and Unipedal Stance used in multiple studies; DGI, Activities Specific Balance Confidence scale, Dynamic Balance Test, Balance Walk used in only 1 study; few studies indicated or demonstrated that the measures were valid for population; one of the included studies validated measures by identifying specificity and sensitivity based on fall history and found that DGI showed the best sensitivity and specificity for patients with diabetes based on existing cutoffs

| Mazzella & McMillan,[89] 2015 | Cross-sectional (level 3) | 25 healthy subjects performed sural nerve block | PS measured before and after bilateral sural nerve block; primary outcome was sway velocity during unilateral stance (4 values, with and without vision under each leg) with 6 additional secondary outcomes (3 PS and 3 tandem walk) | Gait laboratory | Compare stability with and without nerve block | Only unilateral sway on the nondominant leg with eye closed was significantly affected by nerve block; in tandem walk no differences were seen between conditions; sural nerve does not contribute to postural stability |

Abbreviations: ADL, activities of daily living; BBS, Berg Balance Scale; CI, confidence interval; DGI, dynamic gait index; DPN, diabetic peripheral neuropathy; FES-I, Falls Efficacy Scale-International; FFI, foot function index; FoF, fear of falling; FPI, foot posture index; FRT, functional reach test; HV, hallux valgus; LFIS, the Leeds Foot Impact Scale; LLD, limb length discrepancy; MPJ, metatarsal phalangeal joint; OR, odds ratio; PPL, people with lower limb loss; PS, postural sway; RA, rheumatoid arthritis; ROM, range of motion; SLE, systematic lupus erythematosus; TFA, transfemoral amputee; TTA, transtibial amputee; TUG, Time-Up-and-Go; VPT, vibratory perception threshold.

Data from Refs.[24,31–37,46–48,51,77,87–89]

Table 2
Summary of recent studies interventions/experimental comparisons (2014–2019)

Reference	Study Design (Level of Evidence)	Patients	Intervention/ Comparisons	Setting	Outcomes	How Risk Assessed?	Conclusion
Footwear, insoles, and orthotics							
Cockayne et al,[63] 2017; Corbacho et al,[90] 2018	RCT (level 2)	1010 participants (493 IG vs 517 CG) ≥ 65 y old	CG: podiatry treatment + falls leaflet; IG: footwear advice, foot and ankle exercises (30 min/d, 3 ×/wk), foot orthoses	Outpatient podiatry clinic	Primary: incidence of falls in 12 mo Secondary: proportion of falls, QALYs and cost per fall	Prospective falls (baseline, 6 and 12 mo postran domization)	Primary: adjuster IRR = 0.88 (95% CI, -0.73 to 1.05) Secondary: 0.19 falls averted per person-year (95% CI, -0.05 to 0.44) because of intervention; QALY gains in IG not significant; intervention costs £252 more per participant, which amounts to £1253 incremental cost per fall averted

Study	Design	Population	Conditions	Setting	Outcomes	Outcome type	Results
Yick et al,[66] 2018	Crossover (level 3)	5 healthy young adult women; no foot injuries in the past 3 y	6 conditions: 2 midsole × 3 heel heights Midsoles: single forefoot hardness or MHM with hardness Heels: 2, 5, 8 cm	Gait laboratory	Ratio of muscle activation of MG to LG as measure of balance; cocontraction of ankle muscles as measure of gait stability	Changes in listed functional outcomes	Use of the MHM with a 5-cm and 8-cm heel significantly increased the MG/LG ratio during different phases of the gait cycle and cocontraction indices; providing different hardness levels of the midsole material provides more supportive foot–footwear interface
Menz et al,[58] 2017	Crossover (level 3)	30 older adult women healthy, with no injuries in the past 3 mo	Conditions: socks, backless slippers, enclosed slippers	Gait laboratory	Balance (PS, LoS, tandem walk); walking speed, cadence and step length	Changes in listed functional outcomes	Main effects of footwear on all measures with post hoc analysis demonstrating that performance was best with the enclosed slipper and worst with the backless slipper

(continued on next page)

Table 2
(continued)

Reference	Study Design (Level of Evidence)	Patients	Intervention/ Comparisons	Setting	Outcomes	How Risk Assessed?	Conclusion
Paton et al,[65] 2016	Cross-sectional (level 3)	50 patients with DPN	5 insole conditions: no insole, standard diabetic offloading insole, standard with arch removed, standard with cover replaced with memory foam, standard with texture added	Gait laboratory	Standing balance and step reaction time	Changes in listed functional outcomes	There was a significant effect of insole for all but one static balance measure and no effect on reaction time; static balance was significantly worse when participants wore the standard diabetic and memory foam insoles; providing offloading insoles, with arch fill could increase instability; textured cover seems to counter the negative effect of an arch fill
Büyükturan et al,[64] 2018	Cross-sectional (level 3)	56 older adults, with 1+ falls in the past year	Conditions: barefoot, wearing shoes without insoles, and shoes with medium density Plastazote insoles of 5, 10, and 15 mm	Gait laboratory	PS and RoF as provided by the Biodex Balance System	Changes in listed functional outcomes	Across all measure of PS and RoF (static/ dynamic) the best values were observed with the 10-mm insole; for older adults, 10-mm-thick insoles made of medium-density Plastazote may be recommended

					Feasibility	Prospective	
Wylie et al,[62] 2017	RCT (level 2)	43 patients in 6 care homes, with foot problems and history of falling	CG: podiatry care IG: foot orthoses, footwear assessment, and foot and ankle modified exercise program	Care home	Feasibility (retention and adherence) Number of falls, time of first fall	Prospective falls (baseline, end of the 3-mo intervention, after 3 mo, after 6 mo)	Time to first fall for IG was 91 d and CG was 64 d (P = .41); 49 total falls over 9 mo in IG vs 48 in CG but there was a small-to-medium effect size in favor of the IG at 3 mo; between recruitment and study a total of 11 residents dropped out; no adverse events were reported
Yalla et al,[14] 2014	Crossover (level 3)	30 ambulatory older adults (>65 y)	Conditions: barefoot, shoes with and without AFO	Gait laboratory	Functional reach, TUG, balance test	Changes in listed functional outcomes	AFO reduced postural sway with and without vision; no effect on TUG or functional reach
Menz et al,[67] 2017	Cross-sectional (level 3)	30 older women, aged 65–83	Conditions: flexible footwear (minimalistic shoe (Dunlop Volley, Pacific Brands, Australia), commercial footwear (Vigor, Dr Comfort) with a modified outsole to reduce slipping and a modified textured insole	Gait laboratory	PS, LoS, tandem walking, gait (cadence, step length and width)	Changes in listed functional outcomes	No effect of footwear on PS, LoS, or gait; prototype shoes allowed for a reduction of the step width and sway in tandem walk

(continued on next page)

Table 2
(continued)

Reference	Study Design (Level of Evidence)	Patients	Intervention/ Comparisons	Setting	Outcomes	How Risk Assessed?	Conclusion
Wang et al,[68] 2019	RCT (level 2)	44 older adults with concerns of or at risk if falling	CG: fitted walking shoes IG: walking shoes + bilateral custom made AFO	Gait laboratory	Balance (sway of COM, ankle, and hip), physical activity, fear of falling (FES-I)	Changes in listed functional outcomes	Bilateral custom-made AFO plus walking shoes is effective in improving PS and fear of falling compared with walking shoes alone
Exercises							
Martínez-Jiménez et al,[69] 2019	RCT (level 2)	48 young and middle-aged healthy adults	Single bout of continuous vs intermittent stretching of plantar flexors	Outpatient Clinic	PS (with and without vision) and plantar pressure	Changes in listed functional outcomes immediately following stretching	Intermittent stretching of the ankle plantar flexors was found to be more effective than continuous stretching for the reduction of rearfoot maximum pressure and improved 1 measure of PS

Blain et al,[91] 2019	Pre/post intervention (level 3)	134 older adults	Multifactorial assessment of fall risk, which included: 40 min of balance, muscle strength, and functional assessment; 40 min of OT assessment; 20 min podiatrist assessment; 60 min assessment by geriatrician; physiologic testing; followed by patient-specific prescription, which could include physiotherapy or physical activity promotion programs, vitamin D, and podiatric care	Falls clinic	Number of serious fall-related injuries	Prospective falls (recall of 6 mo previous the initiation of the study and 6 mo after)	Serious injuries decreased significantly after 6 mo; fall-related injuries were reduced from 45% to 14.5%; rate of faller from 95.4% to 32.1%, and fear to fall was reduce significantly

(continued on next page)

Table 2
(continued)

Reference	Study Design (Level of Evidence)	Patients	Intervention/ Comparisons	Setting	Outcomes	How Risk Assessed?	Conclusion
Debridement and standard care							
Araguas Garcia & Corbi Soler,[70] 2018	Pre/post intervention (level 3)	48 older adults with plantar hyperkeratoses	Debridement of painful plantar hyperkeratosis	Clinic	Pain and PS	Changes in listed outcomes	Significant pain reduction after intervention; only 2 of 24 PS measures, both in AP direction with vision, significantly improved
Yamashita et al,[75] 2019	Case control (level 2)	180 older adults with foot problems (74 IGs eparated by level of eligible support care; 106 CG matched by age, sex, and support level)	CG: nothing IG: foot and toe nail care (1 ×/mo for 5 mo)	Senior center and podiatry care clinic	Muscle strength (toe-gap, and knee-gap force), foot pressure distribution while standing	Changes in listed outcomes	Knee-gap strength significantly improved for all IG subgroups and toe gap strength improved for 2 of 3 subgroups; pressure distribution improved for all IG subgroups but also for the CG; regular foot and toenail care can improve lower-limb muscle strength

Neuropathy-specific

Kang et al,[79] 2019	Single-arm intervention (level 3)	30 adults with DPN symptoms	Micromobile foot compression device in the shoe insole worn	Community	VPT, SPP, ABI, lower extremity edema, and motor performance (PS and gait)	Changes in listed outcomes	Improvement in VPT, certain measures of PS with and without vision, and certain spatiotemporal gait measures; no significant improvement in SPP, ABI, or edema
Najafi et al,[78] 2017	Double blind RCT (level 2)	28 patients with diabetes and DPN	SENSUS electrical stimulating insole provided to be worn for 1 h daily for 6 wk daily plantar stimulation (SENSUS [NeuroMetrix Inc, Waltham, MA, USA]) CG: placebo, electrical stimulator inactive IG: stimulator active	Gait laboratory Community	VPT, ABI, depression frailty, FES-I, PS with and without vision, gait	Changes in listed outcomes	IG: significant reduction of 27% in VPT (no report of effect on CG), reduction of ankle sway with and without vision (absent in CG), significant increase in cadence (CG group as well) stride length and velocity and significant decrease in stride time (CG as well); no significant changes in ABI or other health measures

(continued on next page)

Table 2
(continued)

Reference	Study Design (Level of Evidence)	Patients	Intervention/ Comparisons	Setting	Outcomes	How Risk Assessed?	Conclusion
HV-specific							
Gur et al,[74] 2017	Intervention (level 3)	18 middle-aged women with bilateral HV	All participants were provided taping corrections	Intervention: clinic Assessment: gait laboratory	5 measures of balance from the Balance Master: mCTSIB, unilateral stance, LoS, step up/over, and walk across tests	Compare balance with and without taping	After taping, HV angle improved significantly; no significant differences between tape and no-tape were found on any of 5 outcomes from mCTSIB, but some dynamic balance was improved after taping (1 of 5 LoS measures and 1 of 2 step up/over); walk across showed increased step width, suggesting taping for HV may impair balance

Prosthetic interventions for amputees

Study	Study type	Participants	Intervention	Setting	Outcomes	Falls outcome	Results
Schafer et al,[84] 2018	RCT (level 2)	15 patients with lower limb amputees (TTA = 5, TFA = 10)	CG: no exercise IG: 12-wk circuit-style group exercise, twice weekly + once a wk at home focused on gait endurance, flexibility, strength, and balance	University	Fall incidence, temporal-spatial gait parameters, and joint kinetics	Falls history (recall 2 y previous study enrollment, and 12 mo after enrollment)	The IG reported fewer falls per person than CG during the 12-mo follow-up ($P = .014$); CG significantly improved walking speed over time but CG did not
Rosenblatt & Ehrhardt,[11] 2017	Case-control (level 3)	27 TTA or TFA amputees (TTA = 15, TFA = 12)	Vacuum-assisted socket suspension (n = 15) vs other forms of suspension (n = 12)	Survey	Incidence of falls and stumbles, rate of falls/stumbles, balance confidence and mobility	Prospective falls (12 mo, recall of every 2 wk)	Although the use of VASS did not affect the rate of falling for either TTA or TFA, the absolute risk of having multiple falls was reduced by nearly 75% in the TTA group by using VASS
Pickle et al,[80] 2019	Cross-sectional (level 3)	20 participants (10 unilateral TTA)	Conditions: walking on a 16-foot ramp at 0°, ± 5°, ±10°; TTA used passive and active prostheses	Gait laboratory	Contributions of arms, legs, and trunk to whole-body angular momentum	Comparing outcomes across between control and TTA using passive and active devices	The trunk and prosthetic-side leg contributions to whole-body angular momentum at toe-off were more similar to nonamputees when amputees use an active vs a passive prosthesis

(continued on next page)

f-

Table 2
(continued)

Reference	Study Design (Level of Evidence)	Patients	Intervention/ Comparisons	Setting	Outcomes	How Risk Assessed?	Conclusion
Shell et al,[81] 2017	Cross-sectional (level 3)	8 unilateral TTA	3 different levels of prosthetic ankle stiffness used during walking around a circular track	Gait laboratory	Walking mechanics (joint kinetics and kinematics), dynamic balance (whole-body angular momentum)	Comparing outcomes across stiffness levels	ML balance improved with decreased stiffness; adaptations in gait mechanics in the coronal-plane were less systematic than other planes; effects of stiffness varied depending on if the residual limb was on the inside or outside; actively adjusting stiffness to turn may be beneficial

Kent et al,[82] 2017	Randomized crossover (level 3)	22 unilateral TTA	2 different prosthetic feet: 1 of an activity level similar to their level (higher activity foot) and 1 rated at a lower activity level (lower activity foot)	Gait laboratory	Margin stability (MOS) in ML and AP directions (COM movement in relation to BOS) measured after initial fitting and 3 wk late	Changes in outcome measure across prosthetic feet	After 3 wk of using the higher activity component, MOS ML decreased on the prosthetic side, and increased on the sound side; similar changes were not seen with lower activity foot where MOS ML was higher on the prosthetic side at 0 and 3 wk; for both feet MOS AP was significantly lower at 3 wk compared with 0 wk; balance changes during walking can occur rapidly after receiving a device; work is needed to determine what these changes mean for function

(continued on next page)

Table 2
(continued)

Reference	Study Design (Level of Evidence)	Patients	Intervention/ Comparisons	Setting	Outcomes	How Risk Assessed?	Conclusion
Wong et al,[85] 2016	Systematic review (level 1)	8 articles that included prosthesis users with TTA	Exercise programs; supervised walking; specific muscle strengthening; and balance, gait, and functional training			Changes in gait speed	Overall there was a low quality of evidence to support the use of exercise programs to improve walking speed in this population; the combined evidence does suggest exercises have the potential to improve self-selected gait speed but additional high-quality research is needed
Other							
Morasiewicz et al,[76] 2018	Retrospective cohort study (level 3)	47 patients who underwent ankle arthrodesis	Group 1: 21 patients who underwent arthrodesis with external stabilization with Ilizarov fixator Group 2: 26 with internal stabilization with screw	Record review	Balance and distribution of lower limb loads using Zebris pedobarographic platform	Between-group comparison of outcomes	Regardless of fixation type, no significant between-limb differences in loading; average loads in each limb were similar for the two fixations; Group 1 had worse balance demonstrated by significantly greater COG area, but similar COG path lengths between groups

| Liddle et al,[86] 2018 | 15 allied health professionals | In-depth qualitative interviews of allied health professionals regarding experiences with interactive fall-prevention training workshops | The first step to a successful program is to value fall prevention in the health care practice; second, it is important to recognize the complexity of multifactorial risk factors and comorbidities assessment; third, one must consider the complexities of integrating fall prevention into routine practice; lastly, adopting strategies for integrating fall prevention in the routine practice is critical; routinizing fall prevention strategies in patient interaction is feasible |

Abbreviations: ABI, ankle brachial index; AFO, ankle-foot orthoses; CG, control group; CI, confidence interval; COG, center of gravity; COM, center of mass; DPN, diabetic peripheral neuropathy; FES-I, Falls Efficacy Scale International; HV, hallux valgus; IG, intervention group; IRR, incident rate ratio; LG, lateral gastrocnemius; LoS, limits of stability; mCTSIB, modified clinical test of sensory interaction and balance; MG, medial gastrocnemius; MHM, multiple hardness midsole; ML, medio-lateral; MOS, margin of stability; OT, occupational therapist; PS, postural sway; QALYs, quality-adjusted life years; RCT, randomized control trial; SPP, skin perfusion pressure; TFA, transfemoral amputee; TTA, transtibial amputee; TUG, Timed-Up-and-Go; VASS, vacuum assisted socket suspension; VPT, vibratory perception threshold.

Data from Refs. 11,14,58,62,64–70,74–76,78–82,85,86,90

oot pain.[22] In addition to the psychological burden introduced by pain, foot pain is particularly problematic with regard to falls because it may impair balance and functional ability.[23] In a study of 135 community-dwelling older people, Menz and Lord[23] found that older people with foot pain performed worse in a leaning balance test, stair ascent and descent, an alternate step test and a timed 6-m walk. Although other foot problems and deformities were also associated with impaired function, in regression analyses, pain was the only independent predictor of all outcome measures. Surprisingly, the prevalence of foot pain was not associated with any specific foot problem, with potential explanations discussed by the authors. In 2018, Muchna and colleagues[24] analyzed data on 128 adults age 65 years and older that were included in the National Institutes of Health–funded Arizona Frailty Cohort Study and found that the odds of having a fear of falling were significantly higher in the 19% of participants who reported severe foot pain relative to older adults with no foot problems (pain, peripheral neuropathy [PN], or deformity); importantly, fear of falling is known to increase the risk of future falls.[25] (Although it is outside of the scope of this review to discuss interventions specific to fear of falling, the existence is worth noting; multicomponent interventions that included exercises for balance, gait, or strength in combination with cognitive behavioral therapy have been shown to be effective for reducing fear of falling and preventing falls in older adults.[26] Here at the Dr. William M. Scholl College of Podiatric Medicine, we are developing similar programs to address the needs of lower extremity amputees[27]). Muchna and colleagues[24] further reported that foot pain increased the odds of frailty and weakness, both of which are known to increase fall risk.[28,29] Surprisingly, the study did not observe a significant increase in the odds of falling with severe foot pain, which is in contrast to a 2006 study by Menz and colleagues[30] that found disabling foot pain predicted falls independent of multiple other risk factors or FA characteristics. The absence of significant findings by Muchna may reflect a smaller sample size, shorter tracking period, and/or different definition for severe/disabling pain. Nonetheless, given the impact of foot pain on functional measures it is important to ask about pain not only with regard to fall risk assessment but with regard to a patient's overall well-being.

When taking patient medical history with a focus on fall risk assessment, it is also important to enquire about a patient's preexisting medical conditions, because many health problems and their associated conditions may increase fall risk. For example, recent studies in our search found that:

- Adult women with rheumatoid arthritis have greater foot impairment and disability than control subjects (as per the Leeds Foot Impairment), and that in this population foot impairments but not pain are associated with a greater fear of falling.[31]
- 26% of individuals who have Parkinson disease and 30% of individuals who survived a stroke self-report having foot problems that influenced their balance; across all subjects, those with a history of falls over the past year were more likely to have foot problems in general and foot problems that influenced balance.[32]
- Common foot problems including corns are evident in patients with systemic lupus erythematosus, with 41% of participants self-reporting currently having a corn or callus. In addition, 27% of persons surveyed self-reported that they would like to "receive footwear advice." Most directly related to falls, "a number of participants [with systemic lupus erythematosus] reported falls as a consequence of altered sensation in their feet."[33]

- Individuals who have survived a stroke demonstrate significantly greater foot pronation than control subjects, as determined by the Foot Posture Index Score, and stroke patients with a history of falls have greater pronation than those who have not fallen.[34]
- The odds of falling for individuals with lower limb amputation and with concurrent vascular comorbidities are nearly 3.5 times greater than for those without comorbidities, even after accounting for amputation cause,[35] with falls being particularly common during rehabilitation.[36]

A 2018 case-control study by Aprile and colleagues[37] provides additional insight into the extent to which amputation may impact fall risk, focusing specifically on patients with foot amputation. The authors compared gait biomechanics (and pain and quality of life) among six subjects with diabetes with first ray amputation (ages 60–90), six subjects with diabetes and no amputation (65–73 years of age), and six healthy control subjects (63–74 years of age). They found that the group with amputation displayed significantly slower walking speed and wider and shorter steps, gait characteristics thought to reflect compensatory strategies for instability (eg, see Ref.[38]).

Note that the bulleted list and study by Aprile and colleagues[37] discussed previously consider only those medical conditions mentioned in articles meeting our search criteria. Podiatrists are encouraged to review the literature regarding other conditions that may be relevant for fall risk assessment, such as obesity[39,40] or osteoporosis.[41]

In addition to the aforementioned medical conditions, diabetes is a particularly important condition for the podiatrist to consider when assessing falls. Indeed, a 2016 meta-analysis found that patients with diabetes are up to 64% more likely to fall than those without diabetes.[42] Although impaired balance and increased falls in patients with diabetes is often assumed to reflect impaired sensation because of diabetic PN (DPN), there is a growing body of evidence to suggest that diabetes, in and of itself, impacts sensorimotor and cognitive process (eg, executive functioning) necessary for balance.[43] When treating a patient with diabetes it is critical that the podiatrist stress the importance of tight glycemic control, not only to ensure overall health, but also to prevent falls. In a cohort of 168 patients aged 60 years or older with diabetes, the presence of hypoglycemia was associated with falls in the prior year and increased the odds of having multiple falls by 360% (95% confidence interval [CI] on odds ratio, 1.2–10.5); the prevalence of falls increased with the frequency of hypoglycemic episodes.[44] Similarly, insulin-treated patients with diabetes are at even higher risk of falling (RoF) than those with diabetes alone.[42]

Finally, when taking a medical history with a focus on fall risk assessment, note a patient's medications. In 2001, Smith[45] examined the top 200 drugs prescribed in the prior year. On eliminating duplicate drugs based on brand and generic names, 169 medications were reviewed. The study found that 9.5% of the reviewed medications had documented adverse effects of traumatic injuries and falls. Thus, as podiatrists it is important to be aware of the extent to which medications may impact patients' fall risk and, when possible, consider alternative medications for patients deemed at high risk based on other factors including those discussed in this section.

Assessing Risk Factors Through Physical Examination

When conducting a lower extremity examination with an emphasis on fall prevention, it is important to be aware of specific foot biomechanics that could impact fall risk. For instance, in 2014, Chen and colleagues[46] found that adults (21–44 years of age) with mechanical ankle instability, but not functional ankle instability, had impaired balance, that is, increased postural sway in the anterior direction when vision is removed, compared with a group of adults free from a history of ankle sprains and other criteria that defined ankle instability. Additionally, Koura and colleagues[47] reported that individuals with bilateral flat feet (n = 20 with >10 mm of navicular drop on the Navicular Drop Test) had significantly worse dynamic balance (higher overall stability index using the Biodex Balance System) at high (but not low) levels of challenge, compared with a group (n = 20) with normal feet. Although this study did not report on falls, and to our knowledge indices from the Biodex Balance System have not been associated with prospective or retrospective falls, a relationship between stability and falls is logical. A 2015 cross-sectional study by Saghazadeh and coworkers[48] provides additional insight into the association between flat feet and fall-risk factors. This study recruited 140 community-dwelling women age 65 years or older and evaluated sitting and standing navicular height and foot mobility (amount of vertical navicular excursion between the positions of the subtalar joint) and postural stability (PS; total path length and area of the center of pressure during a single 30-second trial standing on a force plate). After grouping participants into categories of low, medium, and high arch/mobility, a significant linear trend existed between measures of sway and sitting arch height and between path length and foot mobility with post hoc tests revealing that path length was significantly greater (worse postural control) in older women with low versus high arches. Thus "sitting navicular height may be an important factor in defining balance control in older adults."

In addition to considering foot biomechanics when focusing on fall risk, it is also important to consider foot problem and deformities. In a seminal study on fall risk published in the *New England Journal of Medicine*, Tinetti and colleagues[49] tracked falls over a 1-year period in 336 community-dwelling adults age 75 and older and reported that the odds of falling was 80% higher (95% CI on odds risk, 1.0–2.1) in persons that reported the presence of a severe bunion, toe deformity, ulcer, or deformed nail, after adjusting for sedative medications and cognitive functioning. A separate prospective study on 979 rural, community-dwelling older adults confirmed that bunions can impact fall risk; the presence of bunions in women resulted in a 40% increase in the RoF but doubled the odds of having a major fall-related injury, even after accounting for sedative use.[50] When evaluating foot problems, it may be important to address foot problems that may be specific to a patient's medical history. For example, if a patient presents with a history of stroke one should specifically examine for stroke-related foot problems, including altered sensation, and foot drop, predominantly on the stroke-affected side.[51] Foot drop reduces toe clearance, which has specifically been associated with an increased risk of tripping over obstacles during gait.[9,52] Moreover, in addition to impacting balance, reduced sensation can impact reactive balance strategies once a trip occurs[53]; such strategies are critical to avoiding a fall after hitting an obstacle.[40,54] Impaired foot sensation, specifically PN, is also associated with fear of falling and frailty. Specifically, 42% of participants in the prior mentioned study by Muchna and colleagues[24] had PN (vibratory perception threshold [VPT] >25 V or nonresponsiveness to 10-g monofilament test), and these individuals walked significantly slower and less often than those with no foot problems. Moreover, the odds ratios (95% CI) for frailty and for fear of falling (scores on the Fall Efficacy Scale International [FES]-I) were 13.3 (14–132) and 5.9 (1.8–19), respectively, for older adults with PN compared with those with no foot problems.[24] It is worth noting that in patients with diabetes, who tend to report high levels of falling concerns, the level of neuropathy (VPT) is not associated with the level of fear of falling (FES-I score),[15] suggesting that PN may differently impact patients with and without diabetes.

In addition to examining a patient's foot for problems and deformities when assessing fall risk, it is also important to examine the patient's shoes. The idea that footwear can impact fall risk was best summarized in a review by Menz and Lord,[55] which broadly concluded that:

- High-heeled, narrow-heeled, or open-heeled shoes and slippers may increase fall risk.
- A soft, easily deformable heel counter may increase fall risk.
- Thick, soft materials in midsole construction may cause instability by reducing afferent feedback from the sole of the foot.
- Shoes with a low coefficient of friction could be hazardous but excessive slip resistance may also cause instability under certain conditions.

Accordingly, the authors recommend the use of "…low heels; a fastening mechanism, such as laces, hook and loop fastener, or buckles; flexibility across the metatarsophalangeal joints; a rigid shank; nonslip soles; and a rigid heel counter." Despite these recommendations, patients may prioritize comfort and appearance over safety when choosing footwear. For example, in a sample of 107 persons admitted to a hospital with a fall-related hip fracture, the patients were most commonly (33%) wearing slippers and 73% reported that the footwear they used when they fell was chosen for comfort; only 19% chose the footwear for safety.[56] Similarly, a study that evaluated footwear in 44 patients in two wards of a subacute aged-care hospital found that 86% used footwear that was likely to increase fall risk (ie, footwear with one or more risk features identified in earlier studies[55]) with many wearing slippers.[57] As per findings in a 2019 study, it is important to consider a patient's medical conditions when evaluating footwear because it may be challenging for patients with conditions that impact the lower extremities (eg, edema or braces) to find safe footwear that also accommodates their conditions.[51] Using our search terms we found no articles within the last 5 years that evaluated the relationship between fall incidence and footwear.

INTERVENTIONS TO REDUCE FALL RISK
Shoe Modifications, Insoles, and Orthoses

Although there is considerable evidence that footwear can impact fall risk, evidence to support use of specific types of shoes to reduce fall risk is less clear. In a 2017 study Menz and colleagues[58] directly compared the effects of different footwear on measures of balance and gait. They recruited 30 women aged 65 to 83 years, each of whom performed a series of balance and walking tests in the laboratory while wearing three different types of footwear: socks, backless slippers with a soft sole, and enclosed slippers with a firm sole and Velcro fastening. The study found that "…indoor footwear with an enclosed heel, Velcro fastening and a firm sole optimizes balance and gait compared with backless sippers, and is therefore recommended to reduce the risk of falling," which experimentally supports their earlier recommendations.[55] Despite these findings, there is still a need for randomized controlled studies to better understand the effect of specific footwear on stability to establish unified recommendations among podiatrists.

A fair amount of effort has gone into studying the role of insoles and orthoses in preventing falls. In 2011, Spink and colleagues[59] conducted a trial in which 305 community-dwelling adults older than 65 years of age with disabling foot pain (foot pain lasting for at least a day within the last month and a response of "some days" or "most/every days" to at least one item on the Manchester foot pain and disability index) and with an RoF (fall history in the last year or a score of >1 on the physiologic profile assessment tool, or a time of >10 seconds on the alternate stepping test) were randomized to a control group (ongoing podiatric care) or a multifactorial podiatric intervention that included the provision of prefabricated foot orthoses in addition to footwear advice and provision, home-based FA exercises, and education. The multifactorial intervention significantly reduced the rate of falls by 36%. Six months after concluding the trial, participants in the intervention group were asked how often (most of the time, some of the time, a little of the time, or none of the time) they wore the footwear and orthoses and how often they engaged in at home-exercises. Adherence to the intervention components (responding "some" or "most of the time") was: 69% for orthoses, 54% for footwear, and 72% for home-based exercise with greater adherence in those that were younger, in better physical health, and had less fear of falling.[60] Accordingly, intervention strategies may need to be refined when considering frailer, high-risk older adults. To some extent the moderate adherence rates are surprising given that most participants (>80%) reported that they were "somewhat satisfied" or "very satisfied" with the footwear and orthoses provided.[61]

A 2017 trial evaluated the feasibility of a similarly structured multifaceted podiatric intervention that also included provision of prefabricated orthotics. The study included 43 residents of care homes for older people, each with a history of falls and one or more foot problems, and found that the multifactorial podiatric intervention reduced falls, with 48% of intervention subjects experiencing a fall during the 9-month trial period in contrast to 71% of control subjects.[62] However, because of the small sample size, as dictated by a feasibility study, the difference failed to reach significance; based on the moderate effect size observed (Cohen d = 0.4) a considerably larger sample size is needed to reach significance. In yet another similar study, in 2017 Cockayne and colleagues[63] compared falls between a group of community-dwelling adults age 65 and older with a history of a fall (last 12 months) or injurious fall (last 24 months) who underwent a multifactorial podiatric intervention (FA strengthening exercise, foot orthoses, new footwear if required, and a falls prevention leaflet) versus patients who simply received podiatry care intended to reduce painful conditions, such as corns, callouses, and pathologic nails. After adjusting for gender, age, and history of falling and treatment center, there was a small, nonsignificant reduction in the incidence rate of falls in the intervention group (incidence rate ratio 0.88; 95% CI, 0.73–1.05; $P = .16$) and the proportion of participants experiencing one or more falls was marginally and significantly lower in the intervention group (adjusted odds ratio, 0.78; 95% CI, 0.60–1.00; $P = .05$). However, a larger effect was seen with regard to reducing the odds of multiple (two or more) falls (odds ratio, 0.69; 95% CI, 0.52–0.90; $P = .01$).[63] Collectively these three studies suggest that prefabricated orthoses, along with other podiatric aspects of fall prevention, could assist in decreasing the rate of falls in the elderly. However, because the interventions were multifactorial, the extent to which prefabricated orthoses alone prevents falls cannot be ascertained and future study is warranted.

In contrast to prefabricated orthoses, our search strategy did not yield any recent studies that used custom orthoses in interventional studies. A 2013 review by Hatton and colleagues[4] included 14 studies evaluating the role of footwear interventions (which included custom orthoses and textured and vibrating insoles, customized shoes, and arch supports) on static and dynamic balance and gait. Based on three studies considering custom orthoses they concluded that "Custom foot orthoses seem to be beneficial to immediate and long-term balance performance and gait; however, it remains unclear what underlying mechanism is driving these improvements."

Whether or not footwear is custom made, one must consider features of the insole (eg, thickness or texture) that could impact effectives with regard to fall prevention. A 2018 publication by Büyükturan and colleagues[64] investigated the impact of insole thickness on balance. They recruited 56 community-dwelling adults age 65 years and older with a history of one or more falls in the prior year, each of whom performed tests on the Biodex Balance System to quantify static and dynamic PS and RoF under five different conditions: barefoot; only shoes; and shoes with 5-mm insole, 10-mm insole, and 15-mm insole made of medium-density Plastazote (Zotefoams Inc., Walton, KY). They found a main effect of insole thickness ($P<.05$) on all but 1 of their 12 outcomes measures (PS and RoF each taken under static and dynamic conditions, each taken in two directions and an overall value of each) with post hoc test revealing that the 10-mm-thick insole increased PS and reduced RoF compared with all other conditions. Thus, the authors recommended that "For older adults, 10-mm-thick insoles made of medium-density Plastazote may be recommended to help them with a better PS and a reduced RoF." A 2016 study by Paton and colleagues[65] provides insight into the impact of other insole design components on static and dynamic balance. Fifty patients with diabetes (average age 71 ± 8 years) and insensitivity of a 10-g monofilament at greater than or equal to one site (of 10 sites bilaterally) were observed during quiet stance (standard postural sway assessment) and when stepping in response to a light under five footwear conditions presented in random order: control (no insole); diabetic offloading insole made of EVA/poron; diabetic offloading insole with arch fill removed; diabetic offloading insole with a low-resilient memory foam cover added; and diabetic offloading insole with a textured surface added. Whereas measures of postural sway were worse in the standard diabetic insole and memory foam insole (both with an arch fill) compared with the control condition (no arch fill), postural sway was not significantly different between the textured insole and flat (arch fill removed) insole when compared with the control condition. The authors concluded that "Current best practice of providing offloading insoles, with arch fill, to increase contact area and reduce peak pressure could be making people more unstable" and that "textured cover counters the negative effect of an arch fill" but "flat, soft insoles maybe the preferable design option for those with poor balance." A 2018 study by Yick and colleagues[66] provides additional insight into how cushioning is used to achieve a balance between foot PS (ie, muscle activation) and accommodation and a preliminary study by Menz and colleagues[67] in 2018 provides further insight into how modifying insoles and footwear can improve balance in adults older than the age of 65.

Similar to foot orthoses, ankle-foot orthoses (AFO) may also improve stability and in turn help to reduce fall risk. In a prospective cohort study of 30 ambulatory adults older than the age of 65 years, PS (body sway) was measured before and immediately after receiving a custom-made AFO.[14] Postural sway was assessed as center of mass (CoM), hip, and ankle sway while standing with and without vision using wearable sensors. In addition, coordination between the ankle and hip during a functional reach task was also evaluated. Postural sway was reduced and lower extremity coordination was improved after provision of an AFO. These findings were confirmed by a randomized control trial (RCT) performed by Wang and colleagues in 2019.[68] In this study, 44 community-dwelling adults age 65 years or older, with a self-reported concern about falling or with a fall in the past 6 months or with a Timed-Up-and-Go of 13 seconds or more, were randomized to either a control group that received a pair of walking shoes or an intervention group that received shoes and bilateral AFOs. Balance was assessed at baseline and at 6 months using body-worn sensors to measure sway during tandem stance with and without vision. FES-I and physical activity were also monitored at these time points. The study found that older adults in the intervention group had reduced body sway with vision at 6 months and a significant reduction in fear of falling. Although physical activity was not significantly improved with the intervention there was a medium effect size (Cohen d = 0.52).[68] Thus, AFOs may improve fall risk factors. However neither of these studies directly quantified the effect of AFOs on fall risk; future high-quality trials are needed that include falls as the primary outcomes to justify provision of AFO specifically to reduce falls.

Foot and Ankle Exercises

We have presented evidence that FA exercises, as part of a multifactorial podiatric intervention, is useful to prevent falls,[60,62,63] but there is evidence that FA exercises alone may also be effective. A systematic review and meta-analysis of eight RCTs (one of which was the previously described study by Spink and colleagues[59]) that evaluated the impact of a variety of FA exercise programs on motor outcomes related to falls (ie, strength, balance, flexibility, and functional ability) reported significant improvements in balance and flexibility (weighted effect sizes d = 0.46 and 0.29, respectively) as a result of these programs.[5] No significant effects were seen for plantar flexor strength or walking performance. Because only two of the included RCTs had falls as an outcome (one being the study by Spink and colleagues[59]), no conclusions could be made regarding this outcome. In 2019, Martínez-Jiménez and colleagues[69] conducted an RCT that provides additional insight into the specific type of exercises that may optimize improvements in balance exercises. Forty-eight healthy adults with "no pain" (32.1 ± 7.6 years) were randomized to perform either a continuous or intermittent stretching exercise. The stretching exercise involved standing on a raised platform with the metatarsal head just proximal to the edge of the platform and then lowering a foot without touching the ground; for continuous stretching the lowered position was held for 2 minutes (presumably on each limb) and for intermittent stretching five repetitions of 1 minute each were performed with intervals of 15 seconds of rest. For both groups stabilometry was used to asses balance with and without vision before and immediately after stretching. Center of pressure sway area with eyes open after the exercise (1 of 10 stabilometry measures quantified) was significantly lower for the intermittent stretching group ($P = .03$), although the analysis did not consider subject-specific pre/post changes or adjustments for multiple comparisons.

General Foot and Podiatric Care

Foot pain is an independent risk factor for falls.[22,23] Accordingly, mitigating pain may, in turn, reduce fall risk. For example, in 2017 Araguas Garcia and Corbi Soler[70] evaluated the effect of scalpel debridement (to the underlying pink skin) of painful hyperkeratosis on balance in 48 adults older than the age of 65 years. Balance was assessed using postural sway measures, including center of pressure sway area, path lengths, and velocity taken with and without vision before and after treatment. Several balance measures were significantly improved after treatment, and pain was significantly lower on a visual analog scale. The authors concluded that "Plantar hyperkeratosis debridement is capable of interfering favorably with sensory afferent inputs, thereby improving control of stability and modifying stabilometric readings in the AP [anteroposterior] component when a subject balances with eyes open." Although an earlier study by Balanowski and Flynn[71] reported no impact of debridement on static balance (measured by a Swaymeter as the amount of displacement at the waist height during standing), all three measures of functional ability that were evaluated (time to ascend and descend eight stairs, step up test, and 6-m test) were significantly improved with treatment.

Another common cause of foot pain is hallux valgus (HV).[72] Corrective taping is a conservative treatment option for HV that has been shown to decrease pain[73] but may negatively impact balance (for HV surgeries see next section). In a 2017 study, Gur and colleagues[74] recruited 18 middle-aged patients (45–64 years of age) with bilateral HV deformity (HV angle >15°) all of whom performed balance tests using a

Balance Master computerized posturography device before and after receiving taping to correct the HV angulation (order randomized). Although they observed no significant effect of taping on static balance measures, several dynamic balance measures were improved. However, performance on the "step up/over test" and the "walk across test" was impaired following taping leading to the conclusion that "taping, as an acute effect, may impair balance in middle-aged adults when walking or ascending and descending stairs."

In addition to treating pain as a means to prevent falls, standard podiatric care in and of itself may also be effective. In a 2019 trial (deemed an RCT by the authors), 74 Japanese adults (age 66–98 years) with foot problem (unspecified) and the ability to walk unassisted were assigned to receive foot and toenail care one time per month for 5 months. These individuals spanned all three categories of care-need that are assigned to individuals to participate in the nursing care insurance system in Japan (ineligible for support, eligible for support, and eligible for long-term care). A control group of 104 adults that was propensity score–matched to the "ineligible for support" subgroup was also recruited. Strength was assessed as toe gap force (clamping force between the hallux and the digitus secundus pedis) and as knee-gap force (strength under the knee) at baseline and 5 months later. All three groups showed significant improvements in knee-gap force after the intervention, and two of the three groups improved in toe-gap strength on at least one side, whereas no changes in any strength measures were observed in the control group.[75] That standard foot care can improve strength is critical for fall prevention given that weakness is a known fall-risk factor.[28,29]

Surgical Interventions

In light of the negative findings regarding taping for HV, it is of interest to evaluate the literature regarding surgical interventions. In a 2013 cross-sectional study, Sadra and colleagues[13] compared spatiotemporal measures of gait and static balance (CoM, hip and ankle sway during standing with and without vision, using wearable sensors) among 19 patients with HV as indicated by "bump" pain for greater than 6 months and HV angle greater than 20° (preoperative group), 10 patients who recently underwent successful bilateral HV surgery via scarf osteotomies (postoperative), and 11 control patients. Measures for the postoperative group were taken 10 ± 2.3 weeks after surgery (range, 4–12 weeks). As expected, patients in the preoperative group tended to have poorer static balance control than the other two groups. Although there was a 29% and 63% reduction in CoM sway for postoperative compared with preoperative patients, results were not significant ($P = .17$ and .14, respectively), with minimum gait changes between groups. In a follow-up prospective study, similar balance and gait measures were taken on 13 independent, community-ambulating adults (45 years of age or older who presented with a chief complaint of "bump pain" and a clinical diagnosis of HV before and 1-year following elective, unilateral HV surgery that required a first metatarsal osteotomy. CoM sway during tandem stance was significantly reduced postsurgery ($P = .04$) as was hip and ankle coordination in the frontal plane during quiet standing ($P = .01$ for both).[7] Taken together the two studies suggest that HV surgery may improve certain aspects of balance, but larger studies are still warranted.

In addition to surgical interventions for HV, our search resulted in two recent articles related to the effect of ankle fusion surgery on limb loading with somewhat mixed findings. In a 2018 retrospective cohort study, Morasiewicz and colleagues[76] compared balance and limb load distribution (using the Zebris pedographic platform) between 24 patients who underwent ankle fusion with external fixation using

Ilizarov device and 31 who underwent internal fixation with screws. All measures were taken at least 24 months after their surgery. Regardless of fixation type, there were no significant between-limb differences in loading, and there were no between-group differences in average loads in each limb. Although those who received external fixation had significantly greater center of gravity sway area ($P = .042$), there were no other differences in static balance observed between groups. Thus, there is no strong reason to prefer either surgery when considering balance. In a gait analysis study, Kerkhoff and colleagues[77] compared joint moments and limb load between limbs in eight patients with painless ankle fusion and found that ankle arthrodesis led to small asymmetries in joint movements during gait, with greater loading of the contralateral ankle.

Interventions Specific for Diabetic Peripheral Neuropathy

With regard to reducing fall risk in patients with DPN, several of the studies evaluated in this review involved external stimulation (electrical or vibratory) to promote increased sensation and balance. In one early RCT, an electrical stimulation therapy provided via an aqueous solution was evaluated over a six week intervention. Participants were randomized to either receive or not receive electrical stimulation during treatment and were blinded to treatment. A monofilament test, VPT, and PS test (using wearable sensors to track CoM and hip and ankle sway) were performed at baseline and again at 2, 4, and 6 weeks; then again at a 6- and 12-week follow-up (not all participants completed the 12-week follow-up). Changes in VPT from baseline were significantly different between the two groups at 6 weeks (VPT reduced by an average of 9.6 V in the intervention group and increased an average of 0.1 V in the control group). In addition the intervention group had an immediate reduction in CoM sway that persisted throughout follow-up and was absent from the control group.[16] Thus, preliminary evidence suggested that low levels of electrical stimulation may be beneficial for reducing fall risk in individuals with DPN. As a follow-up, in 2017 Najafi and colleagues[78] conducted an RCT on 28 patients with DPN who were provided non-aqueous plantar stimulators to be used at home daily for 6 weeks. Again, participants were blinded to group assignment (ie, whether or not the device actually provided stimulation) and measures of balance and gait from wearable sensors were compared between baseline and 6 weeks. Following therapy, VPT was significantly improved in the intervention group and the intervention group displayed significantly improved CoM sway with eyes open (Cohen effect size d = 0.67–0.76); there were no improvements in the control group. In addition, all gait parameters were significantly improved in the intervention group. Thus, it is suggested that "daily home use of plantar electrical-stimulation may be a practical means to enhance motor-performance and plantar-sensation in people with DPN."

Our search also found a 2019 single-arm intervention study providing initial evidence that fall risk could be affected by using a novel insole (Footbeat, AVEX, Grand Junction, CO), which provides a small compressive load to the arch of the foot every 35 seconds. The intention of the insole is to increase blood flow to relieve pain, including pain induced by PN. Thirty adults with DPN were provided the insole for 4 weeks and VPT and motor performance (postural sway with and without vision and gait performance during normal, dual-task, and fast walking), among other variables, were assessed before and after the intervention. There was a small but significant improvement in VPT ($P = .007$; d = 0.33), a significant and medium-sized effect of insole use on CoM sway in the mediolateral direction with and without vision ($P = .020$, d = 0.47; $P = .033$, d = 0.66, respectively), and increased stride velocity for all walking tasks.[79]

Interventions Specific for Patient with Lower Extremity Amputation

In a complete discussion of fall prevention, it is important to consider potential cases that could present to a podiatrist but may be best treated with a referral, specifically lower extremity prosthetic users. There are clear biomechanical changes that are present within this population that may alter fall prevention. For example, a study by Pickle and colleagues[80] in 2018 reported that prosthetic wearers tend to use the legs and trunk differently in the control of whole-body angular momentum compared with control participants. They also reported that when amputees use an active versus a passive prosthesis, the contributions to whole-body angular momentum at toe-off were more similar to nonamputees with the active prosthesis, which could have an impact on fall risk. A 2016 study by Shell and colleagues[81] performed quantitative gait analysis on eight unilateral transtibial amputees during curved and straight path walking using three different ankle-foot prosthesis with differing stiffness profiles to quantify the effects of stiffness on joint kinematics and kinetics and dynamic balance assessed via measures of whole-body angular momentum. Among the many findings reported, mediolateral balance was improved with decreased stiffness.

In addition to prosthetic stiffness the type of foot can also impact dynamic stability. In a randomized crossover study by Kent and colleagues[82] in 2017, measures of walking stability were taken on 22 unilateral transtibial amputees immediately after being fit with a new foot (one designed for high or low activity) and again 3 weeks later. After 3 weeks of using the higher activity component, mediolateral stability decreased on the prosthetic side, and increased on the sound side, possibly suggesting a more medial CoM throughout the entire gait cycle, which was not observed on the other foot. Thus components may rapidly lead to changes in balance during walking. However, as pointed out by the authors, the extent to which measures of stability affect function and falls requires additional work.

One study by Rosenblatt and Ehrhardt[11] in 2017 specifically included falls as a primary outcome to evaluate the impact of vacuum-assisted socket suspension on fall risk. In that study 27 adults with varying levels of amputation (transtibial and transfemoral) were recruited, 15 of whom used vacuum-assisted socket suspension; this form of suspension is believed to provide a more intimate fit, which can improve balance and function.[83] Participants completed electronic survey every 2 weeks for 1 year where they were asked to report on whether they stumbled or fell and the circumstances of the fall. When comparing falls between the groups, the authors found that the absolute risk of having multiple falls was reduced by nearly 75% in the group using vacuum-assisted socket suspension.[11]

Exercise programs for prosthetic users have also included falls as a primary outcome. In particular, in 2018 Schafer and colleagues[84] randomized 15 lower limb amputees who sustained a fall in the past 2 years into a 12-week exercise program focusing on gait endurance, flexibility, strength, and balance, and into a control group that did not engage in exercise. At baseline, participants were asked about their falls over the prior 2 years; falls in the year following enrollment were assessed retrospectively at the conclusion of the year. In addition, quantitative gait analysis was performed at baseline and again after 12 weeks. Participants in the exercise group reported significantly fewer falls in the year following enrollment compared with the 2 years prior, and the effect was large ($P = .02$; d = 1.54).[84] The exercise group also significantly improved walking speed, which confirms a 2016 systematic review by Wong and coworkers[85] that reported that exercise interventions targeting speed as outcome for lower limb prosthetic users have the potential to improve self-selected gait speed.

SUMMARY

We have reviewed studies that focus on information relevant to podiatrists when assessing and intervening on fall risk, highlighting those studies that have appeared in the literature within the last 5 years. We refrain from providing specific clinical recommendations based on the literature, because the primary intention is to provide sufficient knowledge to the practitioner to inform their own practice. However, in recognizing the number of methodologies used in the field to quantify balance, we recommend that the field adopt a gold standard for assessing balance in research studies. In addition, we see a need for more high-quality studies with falls as a primary outcome to better inform clinical practice. With that said, if a podiatrist plans to incorporate fall prevention strategies into practice, it is critical to recognize the importance of and process for ensuring buy-in from all relevant stakeholders, to maximize success.[86]

DISCLOSURE

The authors have nothing to disclose.

REFERENCES

1. Bergen G. Falls and fall injuries among adults aged≥ 65 years—United States, 2014. MMWR Morb Mortal Wkly Rep 2016;65:993–8.
2. Center for Disease Control and Prevention. Algorithm for fall risk screening, assessment, and intervention. Center for Disease Control and Prevention, National Center for Injury Prevention and Control; 2017. Available at: https://www.cdc.gov/steadi/materials.html. Accessed January 13, 2020.
3. Najafi B, de Bruin ED, Reeves ND, et al. The role of podiatry in the prevention of falls in older people: a JAPMA special issue. J Am Podiatr Med Assoc 2013; 103(6):452–6.
4. Hatton AL, Rome K, Dixon J, et al. Footwear interventions: a review of their sensorimotor and mechanical effects on balance performance and gait in older adults. J Am Podiatr Med Assoc 2013;103(6):516–33.
5. Schwenk M, Jordan ED, Honarvararaghi B, et al. Effectiveness of foot and ankle exercise programs on reducing the risk of falling in older adults: a systematic review and meta-analysis of randomized controlled trials. J Am Podiatr Med Assoc 2013;103(6):534–47.
6. Crews RT, Yalla SV, Fleischer AE, et al. A growing troubling triad: diabetes, aging, and falls. J Aging Res 2013;2013:342650.
7. Sadra S, Fleischer AP, Klein E, et al. Effects of hallux valgus surgery on balance and gait in middle aged and older adults. J Foot Ankle Surg 2019;103(6): 489–97.
8. Oludare SO, Pater ML, Rosenblatt NJ, et al. Trip-specific training enhances recovery after large postural disturbances for which there is NO expectation. Gait Posture 2018;61:382–6.
9. Rosenblatt NJ, Bauer A, Grabiner MD. Relating minimum toe clearance to prospective, self-reported, trip-related stumbles in the community. Prosthet Orthot Int 2017;41(4):387–92.
10. Rosenblatt NJ, Bauer A, CPO, et al. Active dorsiflexing prostheses may reduce trip-related fall risk in people with transtibial amputation. J Rehabil Res Dev 2014;51(8):14.

11. Rosenblatt NJ, Ehrhardt T. The effect of vacuum assisted socket suspension on prospective, community-based falls by users of lower limb prostheses. Gait Posture 2017;55:100–3.
12. Rosenblatt NJ, Marone J, Grabiner MD. Preventing trip-related falls by community-dwelling adults: a prospective study. J Am Geriatr Soc 2013;61(9): 1629–31.
13. Sadra S, Fleischer A, Klein E, et al. Hallux valgus surgery may produce early improvements in balance control: results of a cross-sectional pilot study. J Am Podiatr Med Assoc 2013;103(6):489–97.
14. Yalla SV, Crews RT, Fleischer AE, et al. An immediate effect of custom-made ankle foot orthoses on postural stability in older adults. Clin Biomech (Bristol, Avon) 2014;29(10):1081–8.
15. Kelly C, Fleischer A, Yalla S, et al. Fear of falling is prevalent in older adults with diabetes mellitus but is unrelated to level of neuropathy. J Am Podiatr Med Assoc 2013;103(6):480–8.
16. Najafi B, Crews RT, Wrobel JS. A novel plantar stimulation technology for improving protective sensation and postural control in patients with diabetic peripheral neuropathy: a double-blinded, randomized study. Gerontology 2013; 59(5):473–80.
17. Najafi B, Horn D, Marclay S, et al. Assessing postural control and postural control strategy in diabetes patients using innovative and wearable technology. J Diabetes Sci Technol 2010;4(4):780–91.
18. Yalla S, Crews R, Khan S, et al. Do objective measures of balance correlate with falls in dementia patients? Arch Phys Med Rehabil 2016;97(10):e96.
19. Cynthia P, Cheng J, Lin F, et al. 'Choose a Game': creation and evaluation of a prototype tool to support therapists in brain injury rehabilitation. In: Proceedings of the 2016 CHI Conference on Human Factors in Computing Systems. Association for Computing Machinery; 2016. p. 2038–49.
20. Lin F, Subramanian V, Swaminathan B, et al. Computer motion gaming provides additional benefits in rehabilitation of mild traumatic brain injury. Arch Phys Med Rehabil 2016;97(10):e130.
21. Dunn JE, Link CL, Felson DT, et al. Prevalence of foot and ankle conditions in a multiethnic community sample of older adults. Am J Epidemiol 2004;159(5): 491–8.
22. Helfand A, Cooke H, Walinsky M, et al. Foot problems associated with older patients. A focused podogeriatric study. J Am Podiatr Med Assoc 1998;88(5): 237–41.
23. Menz HB, Lord SR. Foot pain impairs balance and functional ability in community-dwelling older people. J Am Podiatr Med Assoc 2001;91(5):222–9.
24. Muchna A, Najafi B, Wendel CS, et al. Foot problems in older adults associations with incident falls, frailty syndrome, and sensor-derived gait, balance, and physical activity measures. J Am Podiatr Med Assoc 2018;108(2):126–39.
25. Friedman SM, Munoz B, West SK, et al. Falls and fear of falling: which comes first? A longitudinal prediction model suggests strategies for primary and secondary prevention. J Am Geriatr Soc 2002;50(8):1329–35.
26. Rand D, Miller WC, Yiu J, et al. Interventions for addressing low balance confidence in older adults: a systematic review and meta-analysis. Age Ageing 2011;40(3):297–306.
27. Bourque MO, Schneider KL, Calamari JE, et al. Combining physical therapy and cognitive behavioral therapy techniques to improve balance confidence and community participation in people with unilateral transtibial amputation who use

lower limb prostheses: a study protocol for a randomized sham-control clinical trial. Trials 2019;20(1):812.

28. Ensrud KE, Ewing SK, Taylor BC, et al. Frailty and risk of falls, fracture, and mortality in older women: the study of osteoporotic fractures. J Gerontol A Biol Sci Med Sci 2007;62(7):744–51.

29. Rubenstein LZ. Falls in older people: epidemiology, risk factors and strategies for prevention. Age Ageing 2006;35(Suppl 2):ii37–41.

30. Menz HB, Morris ME, Lord SR. Foot and ankle risk factors for falls in older people: a prospective study. J Gerontol A Biol Sci Med Sci 2006;61(8):866–70.

31. Morpeth T, Brenton-Rule A, Carroll M, et al. Fear of falling and foot pain, impairment and disability in rheumatoid arthritis: a case-control study. Clin Rheumatol 2016;35(4):887–91.

32. Bowen C, Ashburn A, Cole M, et al. A survey exploring self-reported indoor and outdoor footwear habits, foot problems and fall status in people with stroke and Parkinson's. J Foot Ankle Res 2016;9:39.

33. Cherry L, Alcacer-Pitarch B, Hopkinson N, et al. The prevalence of self-reported lower limb and foot health problems experienced by participants with systemic lupus erythematosus: results of a UK national survey. Lupus 2017;26(4):410–6.

34. Kunkel D, Potter J, Mamode L. A cross-sectional observational study comparing foot and ankle characteristics in people with stroke and healthy controls. Disabil Rehabil 2017;39(12):1149–54.

35. Wong CK, Chihuri ST. Impact of vascular disease, amputation level, and the mismatch between balance ability and balance confidence in a cross-sectional study of the likelihood of falls among people with limb loss: perception versus reality. Am J Phys Med Rehabil 2019;98(2):130–5.

36. Hunter SW, Higa J, Frengopoulos C, et al. Evaluating knowledge of falls risk factors and falls prevention strategies among lower extremity amputees after inpatient prosthetic rehabilitation: a prospective study. Disabil Rehabil 2019;41:1–10.

37. Aprile I, Galli M, Pitocco D, et al. Does first ray amputation in diabetic patients influence gait and quality of life? J Foot Ankle Surg 2018;57(1):44–51.

38. Wearing SC, Hennig EM, Byrne NM, et al. The biomechanics of restricted movement in adult obesity. Obes Rev 2006;7(1):13–24.

39. Madigan M, Rosenblatt NJ, Grabiner MD. Obesity as a factor contributing to falls by older adults. Curr Obes Rep 2014;3(3):348–54.

40. Rosenblatt NJ, Grabiner MD. Relationship between obesity and falls by middle-aged and older women. Arch Phys Med Rehabil 2012;93(4):718–22.

41. Patel S, Tweed K, Chinappen U. Fall-related risk factors and osteoporosis in older women referred to an open access bone densitometry service. Age Ageing 2005;34(1):67–71.

42. Yang Y, Hu X, Zhang Q, et al. Diabetes mellitus and risk of falls in older adults: a systematic review and meta-analysis. Age Ageing 2016;45(6):761–7.

43. Hewston P, Deshpande N. Falls and balance impairments in older adults with type 2 diabetes: thinking beyond diabetic peripheral neuropathy. Can J Diabetes 2016;40(1):6–9.

44. Chiba Y, Kimbara Y, Kodera R, et al. Risk factors associated with falls in elderly patients with type 2 diabetes. J Diabetes Complications 2015;29(7):898–902.

45. Smith RG. Fall-contributing adverse effects of the most frequently prescribed drugs. J Am Podiatr Med Assoc 2003;93(1):42–50.

46. Chen H, Li H-Y, Zhang J, et al. Difference in postural control between patients with functional and mechanical ankle instability. Foot Ankle Int 2014;35(10):1068–74.

47. Koura GM, Elimy DA, Hamada HA, et al. Impact of foot pronation on postural stability: an observational study. J Back Musculoskelet Rehabil 2017;30(6):1327–32.
48. Saghazadeh M, Tsunoda K, Soma Y, et al. Static foot posture and mobility associated with postural sway in elderly women using a three-dimensional foot scanner. J Am Podiatr Med Assoc 2015;105(5):412–7.
49. Tinetti ME, Speechley M, Ginter SF. Risk factors for falls among elderly persons living in the community. N Engl J Med 1988;319(26):1701–7.
50. Kosk K, Luukinen H, Laippala P, et al. Physiological factors and medications as predictors of injurious falls by elderly people: a prospective population-based study. Age Ageing 1996;25(1):29–38.
51. Donovan-Hall M, Robison J, Cole M, et al. The trouble with footwear following stroke: a qualitative study of the views and experience of people with stroke. Disabil Rehabil 2019;41:1–8.
52. Byju AG, Nussbaum MA, Madigan ML. Alternative measures of toe trajectory more accurately predict the probability of tripping than minimum toe clearance. J Biomech 2016;49(16):4016–21.
53. Perry SD, McIlroy WE, Maki BE. The role of plantar cutaneous mechanoreceptors in the control of compensatory stepping reactions evoked by unpredictable, multi-directional perturbation. Brain Res 2000;877(2):401–6.
54. Grabiner MD, Crenshaw JR, Hurt CP, et al. Exercise-based fall prevention: can you be a bit more specific? Exerc Sport Sci Rev 2014;42(4):161–8.
55. Menz H, Lord S. Footwear and postural stability in older people. J Am Podiatr Med Assoc 1999;89(7):346–57.
56. Hourihan F, Cumming RG, Taverner-Smith KM, et al. Footwear and hip fracture-related falls in older people. Australas J Ageing 2000;19(2):91–3.
57. Jessup RL. Foot pathology and inappropriate footwear as risk factors for falls in a subacute aged-care hospital. J Am Podiatr Med Assoc 2007;97(3):213–7.
58. Menz HB, Auhl M, Munteanu SE. Effects of indoor footwear on balance and gait patterns in community-dwelling older women. Gerontology 2017;63(2):129–36.
59. Spink MJ, Menz HB, Fotoohabadi MR, et al. Effectiveness of a multifaceted podiatry intervention to prevent falls in community dwelling older people with disabling foot pain: randomised controlled trial. BMJ 2011;342:d3411.
60. Spink MJ, Fotoohabadi MR, Wee E, et al. Predictors of adherence to a multifaceted podiatry intervention for the prevention of falls in older people. BMC Geriatr 2011;11:51.
61. Menz HB, Spink MJ, Landorf KB, et al. Older people's perceptions of a multifaceted podiatric medical intervention to prevent falls. J Am Podiatr Med Assoc 2013;103(6):457–64.
62. Wylie G, Menz HB, McFarlane S, et al. Podiatry intervention versus usual care to prevent falls in care homes: pilot randomised controlled trial (the PIRFECT study). BMC Geriatr 2017;17(1):143.
63. Cockayne S, Rodgers S, Green L, et al. Clinical effectiveness and cost-effectiveness of a multifaceted podiatry intervention for falls prevention in older people: a multicentre cohort randomised controlled trial (the REducing Falls with ORthoses and a Multifaceted podiatry intervention trial). Health Technol Assess 2017;21(24):1–198.
64. Büyükturan O, Demirci S, Büyükturan B, et al. Effects of using insoles of different thicknesses in older adults: which thickness has the best impact on postural stability and risk of falling? J Am Podiatr Med Assoc 2018. https://doi.org/10.7547/17-085.

65. Paton J, Glasser S, Collings R, et al. Getting the right balance: insole design alters the static balance of people with diabetes and neuropathy. J Foot Ankle Res 2016;9:40.

66. Yick KL, Yeung K-I, Wong DP, et al. Effects of in-shoe midsole cushioning on leg muscle balance and co-contraction with increased heel height during walking. J Am Podiatr Med Assoc 2018;108(6):449–57.

67. Menz HB, Auhl M, Munteanu SE. Preliminary evaluation of prototype footwear and insoles to optimise balance and gait in older people. BMC Geriatr 2017; 17(1):212.

68. Wang C, Goel R, Rahemi H, et al. Effectiveness of daily use of bilateral custom-made ankle-foot orthoses on balance, fear of falling, and physical activity in older adults: a randomized controlled trial. Gerontology 2019;65(3):299–307.

69. Martínez-Jiménez EM, Losa-Iglesias ME, Díaz-Velázquez JI, et al. Acute effects of intermittent versus continuous bilateral ankle plantar flexor static stretching on postural sway and plantar pressures: a randomized clinical trial. J Clin Med 2019;8(1) [pii:E52].

70. Araguas Garcia C, Corbi Soler F. Do plantar hyperkeratoses affect balance in people older than 65 years old? Foot (Edinb) 2018;36:43–8.

71. Balanowski KR, Flynn LM. Effect of painful keratoses debridement on foot pain, balance and function in older adults. Gait Posture 2005;22(4):302–7.

72. Benvenuti F, Ferrucci L, Guralnik JM, et al. Foot pain and disability in older persons: an epidemiologic survey. J Am Geriatr Soc 1995;43(5):479–84.

73. Karabicak GO, Bek N, Tiftikci U. Short-term effects of kinesiotaping on pain and joint alignment in conservative treatment of hallux valgus. J Manipulative Physiol Ther 2015;38(8):564–71.

74. Gur G, Ozkal O, Dilek B, et al. Effects of corrective taping on balance and gait in patients with hallux valgus. Foot Ankle Int 2017;38(5):532–40.

75. Yamashita T, Yamashita K, Rinoie C, et al. Improvements in lower-limb muscle strength and foot pressure distribution with foot care in frail elderly adults: a randomized controlled trial from Japan. BMC Geriatr 2019;19(1):83.

76. Morasiewicz P, Konieczny G, Dejnek M, et al. Pedobarographic analysis of body weight distribution on the lower limbs and balance after ankle arthrodesis with Ilizarov fixation and internal fixation. Biomed Eng Online 2018;17(1):174.

77. Kerkhoff YRA, van Boxtel W, Louwerens JWK, et al. Asymmetries in gait and balance control after ankle arthrodesis. J Foot Ankle Surg 2018;57(5):899–903.

78. Najafi B, Talal TK, Grewal GS, et al. Using plantar electrical stimulation to improve postural balance and plantar sensation among patients with diabetic peripheral neuropathy: a randomized double blinded study. J Diabetes Sci Technol 2017; 11(4):693–701.

79. Kang GE, Zahiri M, Lepow B, et al. The effect of daily use of plantar mechanical stimulation through micro-mobile foot compression device installed in shoe insoles on vibration perception, gait, and balance in people with diabetic peripheral neuropathy. J Diabetes Sci Technol 2019;13(5):847–56.

80. Pickle NT, Silverman AK, Wilken JM, et al. Statistical analysis of timeseries data reveals changes in 3D segmental coordination of balance in response to prosthetic ankle power on ramps. Sci Rep 2019;9(1):1272.

81. Shell CE, Segal AD, Klute GK, et al. The effects of prosthetic foot stiffness on transtibial amputee walking mechanics and balance control during turning. Clin Biomech (Bristol, Avon) 2017;49:56–63.

82. Kent JA, Stergiou N, Wurdeman SR. Dynamic balance changes within three weeks of fitting a new prosthetic foot component. Gait Posture 2017;58:23–9.

83. Rosenblatt NJ, Ehrhardt T, Fergus R, et al. Effects of vacuum-assisted socket suspension on energetic costs of walking, functional mobility, and prosthesis-related quality of life. J Prosthet Orthot 2017;29(2):65–72.
84. Schafer ZA, Perry JL, Vanicek N. A personalised exercise programme for individuals with lower limb amputation reduces falls and improves gait biomechanics: a block randomised controlled trial. Gait Posture 2018;63:282–9.
85. Wong CK, Ehrlich JE, Ersing JC, et al. Exercise programs to improve gait performance in people with lower limb amputation: a systematic review. Prosthet Orthot Int 2016;40(1):8–17.
86. Liddle J, Lovarini M, Clemson L, et al. Making fall prevention routine in primary care practice: perspectives of allied health professionals. BMC Health Serv Res 2018;18(1):598.
87. Pratelli E, Alito A, Zanella C, et al. Lower limbs heterometry correction in patients with osteoporosis and increased risk of falls. Clin Cases Miner Bone Metab 2017; 14(3):294–7.
88. Dixon CJ, Knight T, Binns E, et al. Clinical measures of balance in people with type two diabetes: a systematic literature review. Gait Posture 2017;58:325–32.
89. Mazzella NL, McMillan AM. Contribution of the sural nerve to postural stability and cutaneous sensation of the lower limb. Foot Ankle Int 2015;36(4):450–6.
90. Corbacho B, Cockayne S, Fairhurst C, et al. Cost-effectiveness of a multifaceted podiatry intervention for the prevention of falls in older people: the reducing falls with orthoses and a multifaceted podiatry intervention trial findings. Gerontology 2018;64(5):503–12.
91. Blain H, Dabas F, Mekhinini S, et al. Effectiveness of a programme delivered in a falls clinic in preventing serious injuries in high-risk older adults: a pre- and post-intervention study. Maturitas 2019;122:80–6.

Offloading for the Diabetic Foot

Considerations and Implications

Sai V. Yalla, PhD[a],*, Ryan T. Crews, MS[a], Niral A. Patel, MS[b],
Timothy Cheung, MS, CPT[c], Stephanie Wu, DPM, MS[a]

KEYWORDS

- Diabetic foot • Offloading guidelines • Offloading implications
- Limb length discrepancy • Compliance • Foot ulceration • Therapeutic shoes
- Cast walkers

KEY POINTS

- The International Working Group on the Diabetic Foot guidelines for ulcer prevention and ulcer healing are summarized.
- Offloading modalities and their implications, such as limb length discrepancy, lack of compliance, stability, and its effects on the kinetic chain of the lower extremity, are discussed.
- Research at the Dr. William M. Scholl College of Podiatric Medicine at Rosalind Franklin University of Medicine and Science on offloading device design, monitoring activity patterns, offloading device compliance, and gait retraining is reviewed.

INTRODUCTION

The World Health Organization estimates that more than 422 million individuals have diabetes globally.[1–3] In United States, the Centers of Disease Control and Prevention estimates that more than 100 million adults have diabetes or prediabetes.[3] Diabetes has a large spectrum of associated complications with an estimated direct and indirect costs of more than $245 billion.[4] Costs associated with caring for diabetic foot complications constitute a large portion of this financial burden with up to one-third of the total costs for diabetes care being attributable to lower extremity care.[5]

[a] Podiatric Surgery and Applied Biomechanics, Center for Lower Extremity Ambulatory Research (CLEAR), Dr. William M. Scholl College of Podiatric Medicine at Rosalind Franklin University of Medicine and Science, 3333 Green Bay Road, North Chicago, IL 60064, USA; [b] Dr. William M. Scholl College of Podiatric Medicine at Rosalind Franklin University of Medicine & Science, 3333 Green Bay Road, North Chicago, IL 60064, USA; [c] School of Graduate and Postdoctoral Studies, Dr. William M. Scholl College of Podiatric Medicine at Rosalind Franklin University of Medicine & Science, 3333 Green Bay Road, North Chicago, IL 60064, USA
* Corresponding author.
E-mail address: sai.yalla@rosalindfranklin.edu

Clin Podiatr Med Surg 37 (2020) 371–384
https://doi.org/10.1016/j.cpm.2019.12.006
0891-8422/20/© 2019 Elsevier Inc. All rights reserved.
podiatric.theclinics.com

Peripheral neuropathy is highly prevalent in people with diabetes with a lifetime prevalence of 50%.[3] Approximately 19% to 34% of persons with diabetes are expected to develop a diabetic foot ulcer (DFU) within their lifetime.[5] Persistent hyperkeratotic lesions coupled with increased plantar pressure and diabetic peripheral neuropathy are known risk factors for developing DFU.[6,7] Accordingly, offloading areas of high physical stress on the feet is a key tenant to healing active DFU and preventing new wounds.[8] This narrative literature review summarizes recent guidelines for offloading the diabetic foot, discusses challenging implications of offloading interventions, and reviews the work of researchers at the Dr. William M. Scholl College of Podiatric Medicine at Rosalind Franklin University of Medicine and Science to better understand and improve offloading practices.

CURRENT GUIDELINES FOR THE DIABETIC FOOT

The International Working Group on the Diabetic Foot (IWGDF) has recently updated its evidence-based guidelines in 2019 based on systematic reviews and formulation of recommendations by multidisciplinary experts from all over the world.[9] Their recommendations regarding the use of offloading footwear for prevention and treatment of DFU are summarized in this article.

Prevention

Wearing appropriate footwear both indoors and outdoors is a major aspect of prevention, especially in cases of recurring ulceration. IWGDF recommends wearing footwear that leaves at least 1 to 2 cm gap at the toes, with an internal width equal to the foot width, and enough height for all toes. Because individuals with diabetic peripheral neuropathy–induced loss of protective sensation cannot adequately assess fit, footwear should be evaluated by trained professionals. Fit evaluations should preferably be performed later in the day because feet might swell over the course of the day.[10] Extra depth shoes, custom-made shoes, insoles, or orthoses are recommended if off-the-shelf footwear does not fit properly.

Therapeutic footwear with a plantar pressure–relieving effect should be prescribed for patients at high or moderate risk for DFU. Patients at high risk are those with either loss of protective sensation or peripheral arterial disease, and a history of prior foot ulceration, lower extremity amputation, and/or end-stage renal disease. Those at moderate risk have at least 2 of the known risk factors, including loss of protective sensation, peripheral arterial disease, and foot deformity. The prescribed footwear should either have plantar pressure relief of 30% or greater decreases at peak pressure zones of the foot or reducing overall pressure values to less than 200 kPA throughout the foot.[9] These objective offloading targets necessitate the use of barefoot or in-shoe plantar pressure measurement equipment, which may not currently be available to most practitioners. For clinical settings in which plantar pressure measurements are not feasible, it is suggested that therapeutic footwear using available state-of-the-art scientific knowledge be prescribed. In addition to the provision of appropriate footwear, it is recommended that caregivers specifically encourage patients to consistently wear their prescribed footwear whenever possible. Finally, treatment for risk factors such as callus removal, protecting and draining blisters, removal of ingrown toe nails, and antifungal treatments are recommended to aid in the prevention of DFU.

Treatment for Active Wounds

As a first choice for offloading DFU, IWGDF guidelines suggest a nonremovable knee-high offloading device such as the total contact cast (TCC) or an irremovable cast walker, because a lack of compliance is an ongoing issue that deters wound healing.[11,12] If the use of an irremovable device is contraindicated, a removable knee-high offloading device is recommended. In cases where a removable knee-high device is contraindicated or not be tolerated, an ankle-high offloading device is recommended. A large variety of devices were considered to fall under the classification of ankle-high offloading devices, including ankle-high walkers, cast shoes, half shoes, forefoot offloading shoes, postoperative healing shoes, and custom-made temporary shoes. Felted foam in combination with appropriate footwear is suggested as a last choice option for nonsurgical offloading.

IMPLICATIONS OF EXISTING PRACTICES

Although offloading devices help to decrease plantar loading and subsequently contribute to ulcer prevention and healing, it is worth contemplating the potential impact of these modalities on the kinetic chain of the lower extremity and overall well-being of patients that may result from altered gait characteristics, induced limb length discrepancies (LLD), and challenged postural stability. In patients with diabetes, deformities such as equinus[13,14] and hallux rigidus[15] not only increase ulceration risk, but also effect hip joint movement.[16] Moreover, certain offloading devices induce LLD resulting in postural instability and lateral flexion at the L5 to S1 joint, leading to low back pain.[17] Patient compliance with wearing removable offloading devices is suffering owing to these implications.[11] Thus, it might be beneficial for a physician to consider the biomechanical changes of the entire kinetic chain, even when addressing a seemingly physiologic condition.[15,18] These biomechanical implications of preventative and active wound offloading modalities are discussed elsewhere in this article.

Therapeutic Footwear

A prospective multicenter study found custom-made therapeutic footwear (n = 36) have a large effect size of 1.59 (95% confidence interval, 0.57–2.61) of ulcer-free time when compared with standard shoes (n = 33) using multiple linear regression.[19] A randomized controlled study that followed provided custom-made therapeutic footwear, which reduced by at least 20% the peak pressure at high pressure zones of the foot, to 85 patients with diabetic peripheral neuropathy and compared the foot ulceration incidence against a control group of 86 patients with diabetic peripheral neuropathy with usual care non-improved custom-made footwear. Although no significant differences were observed between the groups initially, when the analysis was limited to participants who were highly complaint with their footwear, the plantar pressure optimized custom-made footwear group had a 46% deceased incidence of foot ulceration when compared with standard care therapeutic footwear group,[20] showing the advantages of customizing footwear to patients feet and compliance. Another single-blinded randomized controlled study[21] was performed on 64 controls who received standard orthoses compared with 66 in the experimental group that received offloading orthoses that were designed to address the shape and plantar pressure profile of the foot. Although both standard and experimental orthoses were manufactured using a foam box impression of the participants feet, computer-aided modeling was used to manipulate the impression to achieve a 32% decrease at peak pressure zones of the foot for the experimental group. A hazard ratio of 3.4 (95% confidence interval, 1.3–8.7) for ulceration in the control group was found when compared with experimental group, suggesting that customization of the offloading orthoses decreased ulceration significantly.

When comparing different casting techniques for custom-made orthoses, Guldemond and colleagues[22] found no significant differences in reduction of peak pressures, but gait characteristics varied depending on whether the custom-made orthoses were made as functional or accommodative. Typically, patients with diabetes are prescribed accommodative custom-made orthoses for pressure mitigation purposes. Using in-shoe pressure analyses to guide modifications to custom-made footwear, Waaijman and colleagues[23] showed that peak pressures can be decreased and the decreases can be sustained for at least 1 year. Prescription of custom-made orthoses for the diabetic foot is becoming more prevalent globally as scientific research support grows.[24] Prescription of at least 2 pairs, one for outdoor use and another for indoor use is recommended.[9] This is due to the fact that a high proportion of at-risk patients' daily steps are taken within their homes,[25,26] but adherence to wearing custom-made footwear at home is low.[27] Only 2 studies[28,29] to date have used subjective questionnaires to assess custom-made offloading footwear's effects on gait and stability, which found participants felt they were heavy and difficult to walk in. Although there is strong evidence of decreases of reulceration with the use of accommodative custom-made therapeutic footwear,[30] limited to no attention has been given to study their prospective effects on gait or postural stability, which can be used to toward improving patient compliance.

Total Contact Casts and Removable Cast Walkers

A meta-analysis regarding TCC, irremovable cast walkers, and removable cast walkers (RCW) that assessed clinical benefits and harms, value for money, and patient preference concluded that TCC and irremovable cast walkers resulted in significantly improved ulcer healing in contrast with RCW.[31] This efficacy is secondary to the forced compliance associated with irremovable devices.[12] In 2016, a multicenter trial objectively demonstrated the positive association between adherence in using removable offloading devices and DFU healing.[11] Despite its wound healing efficacy, there are some contraindications and barriers, as listed in **Table 1** that need to be taken into account when deciding to prescribe a TCC.

With these cautions and barriers, physicians may consider RCW as alternative offloading devices. RCW have similar[32] or even higher[33] forefoot plantar pressure decreases when compared with the TCC. However, the removability of RCW strips the reliability of patient compliance. Moreover, owing to the height of the sole of these devices, RCW may induce iatrogenic LLD. Expectedly, patients with unilateral RCW often experience symptoms associated with LLD such as knee, hip, and low back pains, as well as antalgic gait. **Table 2** illustrates select conditions commonly associated with LLD.[34]

One study assessed postural stability, quantified by the degree of sway away from the center of pressure, in a group of high-risk patients with diabetes using various offloading modalities, including TCC with cast boot, TCC with heel, RCW, half shoes, and canvas shoes. The study showed significant instability with TCC with heel compared with all other modalities.[45] Postural stability was also found to be a powerful predictor of noncompliance in a prospective multicenter international study when participants with DFU were monitored for more than 1 month.[11] Induced LLD might be the causality of these postural stability issues that reduce compliance and in turn decrease ulcer healing.

When induced with an LLD of 2 cm or more, Nahas and colleagues[46] found that peak pressure of the total foot on the short limb was increased. The authors also found that peak pressure was higher, specifically below the second to fifth metatarsal heads and that maximum vertical force was increased beneath the third through fifth metatarsal heads, markedly resembling a supinated foot.[46] Thus, physicians must consider the contralateral effects, and the entire kinetic chain, when prescribing

Table 1 Contraindications, cautions, and barriers for TCCs	
Contraindications and Cautions	**Barriers**
Untreated infection or osteomyelitis	Lack of physician skill (improper casting leads to skin
Severe peripheral arterial disease	irritation or even ulcerations)
Deep or heavily draining wounds	Misperception that TCC delays healing
Ataxic patients	Staff training
Blind patients	Cost, time to cast, reimbursement rate
Severely obese patients	Patient reluctance or compliance
	Transportation issues (cannot drive if on right leg)
	Fear of falling
	Storage of supplies
	Assistance in daily activities (ie, bathing and sleeping)
	Cannot use advanced wound-healing adjunctive
	therapies that require daily application
	Cause or exacerbate: deformed nails, ischemia, fungal
	infection, dermatitis, and claustrophobia
	Joint rigidity and muscular atrophy
	Postural instability

unilateral RCWs to heal a DFU, especially if treatment of one DFU may increase the risk of ulceration on the contralateral limb. In an older adult population aged 55 to 68 years with no history of LLD, increased hip and knee flexion, hip abduction, and plantar flexion were observed when induced with 3-cm and 4-cm LLD.[41] The 3- to 4-cm induced LLD resulted in the quadriceps femoris on the longer limb and plantar flexors on the shorter side to compensate with more activity and in turn resulted in increased oxygen consumption and heart rate of the participants.[41] When healthy volunteers were induced with 3 cm of LLD, heel raise gait compensation adapted by participants resulted in asymmetrical lateral bending motion of the spine.[47] LLD can also perturb sagittal plane positioning, where the longer limb tends to pronate with obligatory internal rotation of the leg and thigh, and rotating the pelvis anteriorly. To stabilize against this resultant forward lean caused by pelvic rotation, patients might end up in hyperlordosis, which in turn increases the sacral angle and shear forces at the L5 to S1 joint.[48,49] The lumbar spine and low back pain[50] associated with functional and anatomic LLD[39,40,51] might explain some of the clinical complications observed in the diabetic foot population. Although not specifically researched in participants with DFU, implications to consider owing to congenital, developmental, and induced LLD are shown in **Table 3**.

RESEARCH

Researchers at the Dr. William M. Scholl College of Podiatric Medicine at Rosalind Franklin University of Medicine and Science have substantially contributed to the literature surrounding offloading diabetic feet. This broad portfolio of work can be categorized into 3 themes, namely, physical activity, device evaluation, and foot loading. Although it is well-accepted that the need to offload DFUs is necessitated by physical stresses imparted by the feet during physical activity,[7] the relationship between physical activity and DFU is complex and not fully understood because of issues with compliance, LLD, and stability. We investigated the impact of various offloading device design features on both the capacity of the devices to offload as well as users' experience with the devices. We have also studied ways to help patients with diabetes manage the load they place on their feet.

Table 2
Typical signs of LLD of 3 cm or more and the biomechanical mechanism that causes those signs and symptoms

Signs and Symptoms	Definition	Mechanism
Stress fracture	Focused structural bone weakness developed during the osseous remodeling process occurring owing to repeated above threshold stresses (rate of osteoblast activity slower than osteoclast activity)	Matheson et al,[35] 1987 Muscle weakness decreases the shock-absorbing capability of the lower limb leading, to an increase and redistribution of stress to the bone Friberg,[36] 1982 Force of muscle pull on bone repeatedly exceeds threshold stress Stress fractures in tibia and femur of long limb because there is a tendency to shift weight toward longer limb Langer,[37] 1976 Foot pronation on longer limb to provide functional shortening; muscular stress on tibia increases owing to activation of tibialis anterior as it resists pronation as it nears end range of motion
Functional scoliosis and lower back pain	Transient lateral curvature in those standing with poor posture owing to pelvic tilt in the longer limb First sacral vertebrae is the lowest affected vertebrae[38] First lumbar vertebrae is the most affected vertebrae[38]	Friberg,[40] 1983; Matheson et al,[35] 1987; Giles & Taylor,[39] 1982 LLD-induced scoliosis may cause sciatica on concave side of lateral curved spine and lower back pain as the annulus of the intervertebral disc on the concave side is compressed, leading to dorsal nerve root impingement and the convex side is tensed Gurney et al,[41] 2001 Lower back pain occurred with 3 cm and 4 cm
Secondary osteoarthritis	Thinning and possible perishing of joint articular cartilage Articulating bone surfaces can become thickened or deformed and bony spurs may project into the joint space	Gofton & Trueman,[42] 1971; Maquet,[43] 2012; Radin et al,[44] 1972 Pelvic tilt owing to LLD leads to bilateral unequal knee and hip cartilage and bone stress via increased force and decreased articulating surface area as greater muscle activity is needed to compensate for tilt and there is unaligned bone; during gait, the stresses are increased even more

Data from Refs.[35–37,39–44]

Table 3
Clinical complications observed in multiple studies that researched LLD in various adult populations

Study	Complication(s)
Friberg,[40] 1983; Papaioannou et al,[38] 1982; Blustein & D'Amico,[52] 1985; Danbert,[53] 1988; Gurney et al,[41]; Gofton,[54] 1985; Hoikka et al,[55] 1989	Greater functional scoliosis with greater discrepancy Lumbar convexity on short limb
Friberg,[36] 1982; Fisk & Baigent,[56] 1975; Gofton & Trueman,[42] 1971; Rothenberg,[57] 1988	Longer limb has hip osteoarthritis, hip arthrosis, and hip in a varus position would cause decreased load bearing surface of the femoral head and lead to chondral damage
Rothenberg,[57] 1988	Sciatica in the longer limb Trochanteric bursitis in the shorter limb
Holmes et al,[58] 1993; Subotnick,[59] 1981	Patients with IT band syndrome, which led to knee pain also had an LLD of 0.6–0.9 cm Iliotibial band syndrome occurs in the shorter limbs
Blake & Ferguson,[60] 1992; Gross et al,[49] 2007; McCaw,[61] 1992; Danbert,[53] 1988; Fisk & Baigent,[56] 1975; Gofton,[54] 1985; Kujala et al,[62] 1987	To functionally shorten the longer limb, individuals pronate the foot excessively This leads to internal rotation of the tibia as the talus adducts and plantarflexes and calcaneus everts Internal rotation of the tibia leads to valgus stress on the knee, which could cause medial knee injuries via tensile forces and degenerative conditions laterally via compression stress
Kujala et al,[62] 1987	Athletes with an LLD of ≥0.5 cm had increased overuse knee injuries
Blake & Ferguson,[60] 1992; D'Amico et al,[63] 1985; Resseque & Volpe,[64] 1998; Donatelli,[65] 1987	Severe foot pronation may lead to ankle joint pathology, plantar fasciitis, flat foot, ligamentous laxity, tight Achilles tendon, or hallux valgus, increased weight-bearing force on medial side of the foot
Leppilahti et al,[66] 1998	Achilles tendon was equal in the shorter and longer limb in those with LLD Hence, LLD is not related to Achilles tendon rupture
Friberg,[36] 1982	LLD may cause stress fractures in femur, fibula, and metatarsals

Data from Refs.[36,38,40,42,49,52–66]

PHYSICAL ACTIVITY AND OFFLOADING

Initial forays into objectively studying the association between physical activity and DFU were limited by the technology available at the time.[12,67] Initially, measuring step count was a substantial advancement over subjective reports of physical activity, and presented viable assessment of duration of stress placed on feet over the course of the day. We developed activity monitoring techniques[68] that could differentiate between postural events such as standing, sitting, lying, and walking. A substantial amount of load is placed on the feet during periods of standing, and in the first study to quantify standing time in patients at risk for DFU, we found that participants spent twice as much time standing each day as they did walking.[69] One of the surprising findings of prior investigations regarding the association of physical activity and DFU was that patients at risk for DFU took more steps per day inside versus outside of their homes.[67] This finding was based on merging step counts from a computerized activity monitor with self-report diaries of time spent away from home. Relying on self-reports of locales visited by patients in future endeavors to study the association between environment and physical activity engagement, would leave studies prone to a high risk of both unintentional and intentional errors in reporting. To address this limitation, Scholl College researchers and collaborators from DePaul University developed a methodology for monitoring location-specific physical activity via pairing GPS data with accelerometry-based physical activity data.[25] The capacity to continuously and objectively monitor how physical activity patterns vary according to a person's environment will greatly aid future work addressing the association between activity and DFUs. As discussed elsewhere in this article, compliant use of offloading devices while engaging in weight-bearing activity is a significant challenge to both healing active DFU and preventing new DFU. In 2009, Scholl College faculty in collaboration with the University of Manchester published a methodology for continuously monitoring offloading device adherence through the use of dual accelerometers.[70] This methodology was later used in the multicenter study that objectively demonstrated offloading adherence is positively associated with DFU healing and that self-reported postural instability is a significant predictor of nonadherence.[70]

EVALUATING OFFLOADING DEVICES FOR HEALING DIABETIC FOOT ULCERS

In recognition of the limited use of irremovable offloading devices in clinical practice[71–73] paired with numerous concerns with patient experiences (see **Tables 2** and **3**) using removable devices and subsequent poor adherence with such devices,[11,12] we have investigated how different design features of removable offloading devices influence patient experience with the devices. As noted, the IWGDF recommends using knee-high irremovable offloading devices as the first choice and knee-high RCW as the second choice for the treatment of active DFU.[9] This recommendation is in line with currently available evidence regarding DFU healing. However, knee-high devices are quite heavy, in contrast with standard footwear, and individuals with DFU are commonly physically deconditioned.[74] In a study comparing the functional properties of knee-high, ankle-high, and shoe height RCW, we found ankle-high and knee-high RCW provided similar offloading benefit to the forefoot that was superior to that afforded by shoe height RCW.[75] As a secondary exploratory outcome, that study also evaluated potential changes in gait with the varied offloading options and found a statistically nonsignificant improvement in stability with the use of the ankle-high RCW in contrast with the knee-high RCW. A follow-up study looking at the impact of RCW height on patient experience also assessed a secondary design feature of RCW.[76] Because correction of LLD has been shown to alleviate the symptoms leading to low back pain,[40,77] in addition to investigating RCW size, this study also evaluated the imposition of an LLD by RCW. Walking trials were performed with and without the provision of an external shoe lift for the limb contralateral to the one donning the RCW. This study found self-reported comfort as well as several gait parameters significantly improved in the footwear condition of ankle-high RCW paired with the contralateral lift in contrast with a knee-high RCW with no contralateral lift. The rocker bottom nature of the RCW combined with strut height has also been shown to affect reach velocity and postural stability while reaching for objects. We quantified these metrics in a recent study presented at the American Podiatric Medical Association Annual Scientific Meeting, where ankle-high RCW had better postural stability without affecting reach distance while also decreasing reach velocity when compared with knee-high RCW.[78] We suspect a reduction of reach velocity might help with better control during day-to-day tasks and might help with compliance with these offloading devices. Additional prospective studies are needed to determine if ankle-high RCW paired with a contralateral lift can truly translate into improved adherence and subsequent DFU healing.

HELPING PATIENTS MANAGE FOOT LOADING

Although offloading devices can be used to mitigate the load diabetic feet are exposed to, the volume of activity engaged in and the biomechanical parameters associated with that activity will dictate the magnitude of stress that needs to be accounted for. Although too much loading is unquestionably problematic for diabetic feet, too little activity is also a potential problem.[79–81] In recognition of the difficult balancing act of having patients engage in physical activity in a manner that will help them to manage their diabetes and overall health without inducing a DFU,[81] our group recently published results of a feasibility study regarding physical activity engagement by individuals at risk for DFU.[82] Preliminary evidence indicated that low-intensity, technology-based behavioral interventions resulted in increased walking activity and was well-accepted by study participants. We also investigated the potential to use accelerometer technology to train individuals to reduce the load (ground reaction forces)[83] imparted during walking by providing visual feedback of their tibial acceleration. Participants were asked to manipulate their gait until tibial acceleration was reduced by 25%, and the ground reaction forces did reduce during walking and jogging while also improving symmetry. In addition to assisting with offloading, such training may also help with mitigating device induced low back pain. Visual cues are capable of reducing vertical ground reaction forces by modifying strike pattern, increasing cadence as well as activation of the transversus abdominis and obliquus internus abdominis muscles that help with spinal stability and treat low back pain.[84–86]

In addition to investigating ways to help patients at risk for DFU to safely partake in appropriate levels of physical activity, we have also studied the potential to allow patients with active DFU to safely exercise. In 2008, we published a proof-of-concept trial regarding a cleat for use with stationary bicycles.[87] The cleat was intended to permit exercise using the lower extremities without imparting significant loading to a forefoot DFU. The initial study demonstrated the cleat significantly reduced forefoot loading in healthy subjects in comparison to a standard cleat. A secondary early stage study confirmed the cleat significantly reduced forefoot loading in patients at risk for DFU.[88] This study also found cycling with the device resulted in increased perfusion to the distal portion of feet, which suggests there may be wound healing benefits.

SUMMARY

The diabetes prevalence rate increased by 26% from 2012 to 2018 and it continues to be an economic burden.[89] Offloading remains a cornerstone in the prevention and treatment of the diabetic foot.[9,90] Custom-made accommodative orthoses and therapeutic footwear are effective at preventing ulcer recurrence as long as the patients are compliant in wearing them,[91] but limited attention has been given to their effects on gait symmetry and stability. Offloading devices such as TCC and irremovable RCW have been effective in healing active ulcers, but they induce LLD, which can affect the gait mechanics of the patient, and in turn lead to multiple issues all across the kinetic chain up to the lower back.[18] Addressing these implications might lead to improved compliance that is currently lacking in the diabetic foot population. Using lifts for LLD correction, understanding patient activity patterns using location-specific monitoring, and providing biofeedback via visual cues are some of the innovative ways Scholl researchers are investigating means to improve offloading interventions. Scholl researchers are also contributing to the literature surrounding the diabetic foot by investigating offloading design modifications, monitoring physical activity along with compliance inside and outside participant's home, thereby advancing avenues to improve offloading device compliance. The diabetic foot remains a complex problem, but recent advances toward addressing the implications of existing interventions can create a holistic approach that might be able to prevent and heal ulcers while preserving the whole body gait biomechanics for improving quality of life.

REFERENCES

1. Prem NN, Gupta M, Gupta T. Existing predictive models of diabetes: A review. SF J Diabetes Endocrin 2018;2:2.
2. Juster-Switlyk K, Smith AG. Updates in diabetic peripheral neuropathy. F1000Res 2016;5 [pii:F1000].
3. Control CfD. Prevention. National diabetes statistics report, 2017. Atlanta (GA): Centers for Disease Control and Prevention, US Department of Health and Human Services; 2017.
4. McCall B. Huge burden of foot ulcers doubles diabetes costs in US. Medscape Medical News 2014;13.
5. Armstrong DG, Boulton AJM, Bus SA. Diabetic foot ulcers and their recurrence. N Engl J Med 2017;376(24):2367–75.
6. Amemiya A, Noguchi H, Oe M, et al. Shear stress-normal stress (pressure) ratio decides forming callus in patients with diabetic neuropathy. J Diabetes Res 2016; 2016:3157123.
7. Wu SC, Crews RT, Armstrong DG. The pivotal role of offloading in the management of neuropathic foot ulceration. Curr Diab Rep 2005;5(6):423–9.
8. Bus SA, van Deursen RW, Armstrong DG, et al. Footwear and offloading interventions to prevent and heal foot ulcers and reduce plantar pressure in patients with diabetes: a systematic review. Diabetes Metab Res Rev 2016;32(Suppl 1):99–118.
9. Bus SA, Armstrong DG, Gooday C, et al. IWGDF guideline on offloading foot ulcers in persons with diabetes. Diabetes Metab Res Rev 2019.
10. Reiber GE, Ledoux WR. Epidemiology of foot ulcers and amputations in people with diabetes: evidence for prevention. In: Herman WH, Kinmonth AL, Wareham NJ, et al, editors. The Evidence Base for Diabetes Care. Second Edition. John Wiley & Sons, Ltd; 2010. p. 403–17.
11. Crews RT, Shen BJ, Campbell L, et al. Role and determinants of adherence to offloading in diabetic foot ulcer healing: a prospective investigation. Diabetes Care 2016;39(8):1371–7.
12. Armstrong DG, Lavery LA, Kimbriel HR, et al. Activity patterns of patients with diabetic foot ulceration: patients with active ulceration may not adhere to a standard pressure off-loading regimen. Diabetes Care 2003;26(9):2595–7.
13. Lin SS, Lee TH, Wapner KL. Plantar forefoot ulceration with equinus deformity of the ankle in diabetic patients: the effect of tendo-Achilles lengthening and total contact casting. Orthopedics 1996;19(5):465–75.
14. Searle A, Spink M, Chuter V. Prevalence of ankle equinus and correlation with foot plantar pressures in people with diabetes. Clin Biomech 2018;60:39–44.
15. Dananberg HJ. Sagittal plane biomechanics. American Diabetes Association. J Am Podiatr Med Assoc 2000;90(1):47–50.

16. Dananberg HJ. Lower extremity mechanics and their effect of lumbosacral function. In: Dorman T, editor. Spine: State of the Art Reviews. Philadelphia: Henley & Belfus; 1995. p. 389–405.
17. Thorstensson A, Arvidson A. Trunk muscle strength and low back pain. Scand J Rehabil Med 1982;14(2):69–75.
18. Curran S, Dananberg H. Future of gait analysis: a podiatric medical perspective. J Am Podiatr Med Assoc 2005;95(2):130.
19. Uccioli L, Faglia E, Monticone G, et al. Manufactured shoes in the prevention of diabetic foot ulcers. Diabetes Care 1995;18(10):1376–8.
20. Bus SA, Waaijman R, Arts M, et al. Effect of custom-made footwear on foot ulcer recurrence in diabetes: a multicenter randomized controlled trial. Diabetes Care 2013;36(12):4109–16.
21. Ulbrecht JS, Hurley T, Mauger DT, et al. Prevention of recurrent foot ulcers with plantar pressure-based in-shoe orthoses: the CareFUL prevention multicenter randomized controlled trial. Diabetes Care 2014;37(7):1982–9.
22. Guldemond NA, Leffers P, Sanders AP, et al. Casting methods and plantar pressure: effects of custom-made foot orthoses on dynamic plantar pressure distribution. J Am Podiatr Med Assoc 2006;96(1):9–18.
23. Waaijman R, Arts ML, Haspels R, et al. Pressure-reduction and preservation in custom-made footwear of patients with diabetes and a history of plantar ulceration. Diabet Med 2012;29(12):1542–9.
24. Chapman LS, Redmond AC, Landorf KB, et al. A survey of foot orthoses prescription habits amongst podiatrists in the UK, Australia and New Zealand. J Foot Ankle Res 2018;11(1):64.
25. Crews RT, Yalla SV, Dhatt N, et al. Monitoring location-specific physical activity via integration of accelerometry and geotechnology within patients with or at risk of diabetic foot ulcers: a technological report. J Diabetes Sci Technol 2017;11(5):899–903.
26. Cloix L, Caille A, Helmer C, et al. Physical activity at home, at leisure, during transportation and at work in French adults with type 2 diabetes: the ENTRED physical activity study. Diabetes Metab 2015;41(1):37–44.
27. Waaijman R, Keukenkamp R, de Haart M, et al. Adherence to wearing prescription custom-made footwear in patients with diabetes at high risk for plantar foot ulceration. Diabetes Care 2013;36(6):1613–8.
28. Paton JS, Roberts A, Bruce GK, et al. Does footwear affect balance? The views and experiences of people with diabetes and neuropathy who have fallen. J Am Podiatr Med Assoc 2013;103(6):508–15.
29. Arts ML, de Haart M, Bus SA, et al. Perceived usability and use of custom-made footwear in diabetic patients at high risk for foot ulceration. J Rehabil Med 2014;46(4):357–62.
30. Jorgetto JV, Gamba MA, Kusahara DM. Evaluation of the use of therapeutic footwear in people with diabetes mellitus–a scoping review. J Diabetes Metab Disord 2019;18(2):613–24.
31. Ontario HQ. Fibreglass total contact casting, removable cast walkers, and irremovable cast walkers to treat diabetic neuropathic foot ulcers: a health technology assessment. Ont Health Technol Assess Ser 2017;17(12):1.
32. de Oliveira AM, Moore Z. Treatment of the diabetic foot by offloading: a systematic review. J Wound Care 2015;24(12):560–70.
33. Westra M, van Netten JJ, Manning HA, et al. Effect of different casting design characteristics on offloading the diabetic foot. Gait Posture 2018;64:90–4.

34. Mieras JN, Singleton TJ, Barrett SL. Contralateral peak plantar pressures with a post-operative boot: a preliminary study. J Am Podiatr Med Assoc 2011;101(2):127–32.
35. Matheson G, Clement D, McKenzie D, et al. Stress fractures in athletes: a study of 320 cases. Am J Sports Med 1987;15(1):46–58.
36. Friberg O. Leg length asymmetry in stress fractures. A clinical and radiological study. J Sports Med Phys Fitness 1982;22(4):485.
37. Langer S. Structural leg shortage. A case report. J Am Podiatr Med Assoc 1976; 66(1):38–40.
38. Papaioannou T, Stokes I, Kenwright J. Scoliosis associated with limb-length inequality. J Bone Joint Surg Am 1982;64(1):59–62.
39. Giles L, Taylor J. Lumbar spine structural changes associated with leg length inequality. Spine 1982;7(2):159–62.
40. Friberg O. Clinical symptoms and biomechanics of lumbar spine and hip joint in leg length inequality. Spine 1983;8(6):643–51.
41. Gurney B, Mermier C, Robergs R, et al. Effects of limb-length discrepancy on gait economy and lower-extremity muscle activity in older adults. J Bone Joint Surg Am 2001;83-A(6):907–15.
42. Gofton J, Trueman G. Studies in osteoarthritis of the hip: part II,* Osteoarthritis of the hip and leg-length disparity. Can Med Assoc J 1971;104(9):791.
43. Maquet PG. Biomechanics of the knee: with application to the pathogenesis and the surgical treatment of osteoarthritis. New York: Springer-Verlag Berlin Heidelberg; 2012.
44. Radin E, Paul I, Rose R. Role of mechanical factors in pathogenesis of primary osteoarthritis. Lancet 1972;299(7749):519–22.
45. Lavery LA, Fleishli JG, Laughlin TJ, et al. Is postural instability exacerbated by off-loading devices in high risk diabetics with foot ulcers? Ostomy Wound Manage 1998;44(1):26–32, 34.
46. Nahas MR, Gawish HM, Tarshoby MM, et al. Effect of simulated leg length discrepancy on plantar pressure distribution in diabetic patients with neuropathic foot ulceration. J Wound Care 2011;20(10):473–7.
47. Kakushima M, Miyamoto K, Shimizu K. The effect of leg length discrepancy on spinal motion during gait: three-dimensional analysis in healthy volunteers. Spine 2003;28(21):2472–6.
48. Perry J, Burnfield J. Kinetics of gait: ground reaction forces, vectors, moments, power and pressure. Gait Analysis: normal and pathological function second. Thorofare (NJ): Slack Incorporated; 2010. p. 457–70.
49. Gross KD, Niu J, Zhang YQ, et al. Varus foot alignment and hip conditions in older adults. Arthritis Rheum 2007;56(9):2993–8.
50. Giles L, Taylor J. Low-back pain associated with leg length inequality. Spine 1981;6(5):510–21.
51. Ryan Crews M, Girgis C, Domijancic R, et al. Influence of Offloading Induced Limb Length Discrepancies upon Spinal Alignment. Paper presented at: American Diabetes Association 77th Scientific Sessions2017. San Diego, CA, June 9-13, 2017.
52. Blustein SM, D'Amico JC. Limb length discrepancy. Identification, clinical significance, and management. J Am Podiatr Med Assoc 1985;75(4):200–6.
53. Danbert R. Clinical assessment and treatment of leg length inequalities. J Manipulative Physiol Ther 1988;11(4):290–5.
54. Gofton J. Persistent low back pain and leg length disparity. J Rheumatol 1985; 12(4):747–50.

55. Hoikka V, Ylikoski M, Tallroth K. Leg-length inequality has poor correlation with lumbar scoliosis. Arch Orthop Trauma Surg 1989;108(3):173–5.
56. Fisk J, Baigent M. Clinical and radiological assessment of leg length. N Z Med J 1975;81(540):477–80.
57. Rothenberg RJ. Rheumatic disease aspects of leg length inequality. Semin Arthritis Rheum 1988;17(3):196-205.
58. Holmes JC, Pruitt AL, Whalen NJ. Iliotibial band syndrome in cyclists. Am J Sports Med 1993;21(3):419–24.
59. Subotnick SI. Limb length discrepancies of the lower extremity (the short leg syndrome). J Orthop Sports Phys Ther 1981;3(1):11–6.
60. Blake R, Ferguson H. Limb length discrepancies. J Am Podiatr Med Assoc 1992; 82(1):33–8.
61. McCaw ST. Leg length inequality. Sports Med 1992;14(6):422–9.
62. Kujala U, Friberg O, Aalto T, et al. Lower limb asymmetry and patellofemoral joint incongruence in the etiology of knee exertion injuries in athletes. Int J Sports Med 1987;8(03):214–20.
63. D'Amico J, Dinowitz H, Polchaninoff M. Limb length discrepancy. An electrodynographic analysis. J Am Podiatr Med Assoc 1985;75(12):639–43.
64. Resseque B, Volpe R. Progressive subtalar joint dislocation and limb-length inequality. An unusual case. J Am Podiatr Med Assoc 1998;88(4):176–80.
65. Donatelli R. Abnormal biomechanics of the foot and ankle. J Orthop Sports Phys Ther 1987;9(1):11.
66. Leppilahti J, Korpelainen R, Karpakka J, et al. Ruptures of the Achilles tendon: relationship to inequality in length of legs and to patterns in the foot and ankle. Foot Ankle Int 1998;19(10):683–7.
67. Armstrong DG, Abu-Rumman PL, Nixon BP, et al. Continuous activity monitoring in persons at high risk for diabetes-related lower-extremity amputation. J Am Podiatr Med Assoc 2001;91(9):451–5.
68. Najafi B, Wrobel J, Armstrong D. A Novel Ambulatory device for continuous 24-H monitoring of physical activity in daily life (Abstract#586). North American Congress on Biomechanics (NACOB); August, 2008, 2008, Ann Arbor, MI, August 5-9, 2008.
69. Najafi B, Crews RT, Wrobel JS. Importance of time spent standing for those at risk of diabetic foot ulceration. Diabetes Care 2010;33(11):2448–50.
70. Crews RT, Armstrong DG, Boulton AJ. A method for assessing off-loading compliance. J Am Podiatr Med Assoc 2009;99(2):100–3.
71. Wu SC, Jensen JL, Weber AK, et al. Use of pressure offloading devices in diabetic foot ulcers: do we practice what we preach? Diabetes Care 2008;31(11):2118–9.
72. Raspovic A, Landorf KB. A survey of offloading practices for diabetes-related plantar neuropathic foot ulcers. J Foot Ankle Res 2014;7:35.
73. Quinton TR, Lazzarini PA, Boyle FM, et al. How do Australian podiatrists manage patients with diabetes? The Australian diabetic foot management survey. J Foot Ankle Res 2015;8:16.
74. Kanade RV, van Deursen RW, Harding K, et al. Walking performance in people with diabetic neuropathy: benefits and threats. Diabetologia 2006;49(8):1747–54.
75. Crews RT, Sayeed F, Najafi B. Impact of strut height on offloading capacity of removable cast walkers. Clin Biomech (Bristol, Avon) 2012;27(7):725–30.
76. Crews RT, Candela J. Decreasing an offloading device's size and offsetting its imposed limb-length discrepancy lead to improved comfort and gait. Diabetes Care 2018;41(7):1400–5.

77. Friberg O. Biomechanical significance of the correct length of lower limb prostheses: a clinical and radiological study. Prosthet Orthot Int 1984;8(3):124–9.

78. Arwa Akram. Ann Kim RR, Vasanth Subramanian, et al. Using balance and reach velocity assessments to identify removable cast walker StrutHeight influence on patients with diabetes. 2018. Available at: https://www.apma.org/files/APMA%20Presentation%20Arwa%20Akram.pdf. Accessed September 15, 2019.

79. Lemaster JW, Reiber GE, Smith DG, et al. Daily weight-bearing activity does not increase the risk of diabetic foot ulcers. Med Sci Sports Exerc 2003;35(7):1093–9.

80. Armstrong DG, Lavery LA, Holtz-Neiderer K, et al. Variability in activity may precede diabetic foot ulceration. Diabetes Care 2004;27(8):1980–4.

81. Crews RT, Schneider KL, Yalla SV, et al. Physiological and psychological challenges of increasing physical activity and exercise in patients at risk of diabetic foot ulcers: a critical review. Diabetes Metab Res Rev 2016;32(8):791–804.

82. Schneider KL, Crews RT, Subramanian V, et al. Feasibility of a low-intensity, technology-based intervention for increasing physical activity in adults at risk for a diabetic foot ulcer: a mixed-methods study. J Diabetes Sci Technol 2019;13(5):857–68.

83. Nikita Grama BW, Mahabamunage S, Stanton W, et al. Gait manipulation using visual feedback and its influence on ground reaction forces. 2018. Available at: https://www.apma.org/files/APMA_Visual%20Feedback%20study_NG_SVY_071318.pdf. Accessed September 15, 2019.

84. Unsgaard-Tøndel M, Nilsen TIL, Magnussen J, et al. Is activation of transversus abdominis and obliquus internus abdominis associated with long-term changes in chronic low back pain? A prospective study with 1-year follow-up. Br J Sports Med 2012;46(10):729–34.

85. Selkow NM, Eck MR, Rivas S. Transversus abdominis activation and timing improves following core stability training: a randomized trial. Int J Sports Phys Ther 2017;12(7):1048–56.

86. Barrios JA, Crossley KM, Davis IS. Gait retraining to reduce the knee adduction moment through real-time visual feedback of dynamic knee alignment. J Biomech 2010;43(11):2208–13.

87. Klein EE, Crews RT, Wu SC, et al. CLEAR Cleat: a proof-of-concept trial of an aerobic activity facilitator to reduce plantar forefoot pressures and their potential in those with foot ulcers. J Am Podiatr Med Assoc 2008;98(4):261–7.

88. Crews RT, Smith SR, Ghazizadeh R, et al. Preliminary evaluation of a cycling cleat designed for diabetic foot ulcers. J Am Podiatr Med Assoc 2017;107(6):475–82.

89. Association AD. Economic costs of diabetes in the US in 2017. Diabetes care 2018;41(5):917–28.

90. Bus SA. Offloading the diabetic foot: the evolution of an integrated strategy. In: Piaggesi A, Apelqvist J, editors. The Diabetic Foot Syndrome. Front Diabetes. Basel: Karger; 2018. p. 97–106.

91. Cavanagh PR, Bus SA. Off-loading the diabetic foot for ulcer prevention and healing. Plast Reconstr Surg 2011;127:248S.

VIII. Barry University School of Podiatric Medicine

Lack of Transparency in Publishing Negative Clinical Trial Results

Robert J. Snyder, DPM, MSc, CWSP, FFPM RCPS (Glasgow)*

KEYWORDS

- Clinical research • Negative results • Randomized control trials

KEY POINTS

- Researchers often do not publish negative results.
- Failure to release less than favorable results could be construed as ethically and morally inappropriate.
- Failure to make public less than favorable outcomes stifles the scientific process and is contrary to the precepts of the Declaration of Helsinki and the World Health Organization.
- Sponsors and researchers must embrace the ideal of publishing well-designed studies with negative results.

INTRODUCTION

Clinical research remains the bedrock for finding cures to the most challenging medical maladies. Unfortunately, it is common practice for researchers and sponsors not to publish negative results.

Sadly, failure to release less than favorable results could be construed as ethically and morally inappropriate and could lead to a waste of resources, and potential harm to patients.[1,2] At the very least, researchers and sponsors have an ethical and moral obligation to trial participants who depended on them.[3–7] This is particularly germane when another sponsor is considering going down the same road to a treatment that likely will not work.[5]

Failure to make public less than favorable outcomes stifles the scientific process and is contrary to precepts of the Declaration of Helsinki and the World Health Organization.[8] This even includes a reluctance in sharing results.[9]

Nygaard[10] suggests that sponsors and researchers must embrace the ideal of publishing well-designed studies with negative results. Doing so could protect the integrity of the research process and minimize skewing of the literature while shielding patients

Barry University School of Podiatric Medicine, Miami Shores, FL, USA
* 7301 North University Drive, Suite 305, Tamarac, FL 33321.
E-mail address: DRWOUND@AOL.COM

Clin Podiatr Med Surg 37 (2020) 385–389
https://doi.org/10.1016/j.cpm.2019.12.013
0891-8422/20/© 2019 Elsevier Inc. All rights reserved.

from failed treatments. Additionally, such publications could glean important scientific reflections that may reduce bias and improve drug efficacy while protecting patients.[11] Therefore, sponsors that avoid publishing negative data foster bias, misinformation, and potential harm to future subjects.[5] In a variety of instances, large pharmaceutical companies, such as Glaxo, have published negative results without reservation.[12] However, more often than not, this process remains elusive.

ANALYSIS

Unger and colleagues[11] opined that positive outcome-reported bias remains rampant and there is published validation that reviewers are less likely to recommend disseminating the results of trials with negative results. Irresponsible behavior on the part of pharmaceutical companies by not publishing trials with negative outcomes derails the scientific process and is contrary to precepts of the Declaration of Helsinki and the World Health Organization.[8]

Naysayers continually point to the national and international registries, such as ClinicalTrials.gov,[13] European Union's Clinical Trials Directive,[14] and the World Health Organization's International Clinical Trials Registry Platform,[15] which allow for the sharing of negative trial results and may preclude the need for formal publications.

However, this practice occurs in small numbers. Underreporting and nonpublication of negative results is pervasive.[9] Biased conclusions could detrimentally affect clinical practice, patients, and policy decisions; urgent measures are therefore required to reverse this trend.[5]

Analysis reveals that, with few exceptions, the pharmaceutical industry is notorious for burying negative results largely to protect shareholders and profits.[16] Furthermore, researchers flagrantly fail to publish or even register negative trial results or, worse, alter results to make the data more appealing to journal editors and reviewers.[17] For example, compliance with the European Commission mandate revealed that half of all trials were out of compliance.[18,19] Further, the New England Journal of Medicine reported that only about 20% of trials supported by industry conveyed results on ClinicalTrials.gov and 50% of trials sponsored by the National Institutes of Health failed to report.[20] This is particularly rampant in academia where the "publish or perish" mantra remains the gold standard.[21] It remains clear that publishing negative results, such as the COURAGE trial, disproving that cardiovascular stenting is superior to medical treatment, had a positive impact on patient care.[22] Unfortunately, such studies have historically been underreported.

Although conveying clinical results on registries, such as ClinicalTrials.gov,[13] has been required, discrepancies exist between results provided on the registries and publications, suggesting potential bias and underreporting or nonreporting. This could lead to a lack of validity in the information provided to the registry. The Food and Drug Administration is so concerned about this practice that the agency has initiated a recommendation to garner civil monetary penalties for those entities that are not in compliance.[17] In the European Union, there are similar concerns including the lack in expertise of reviewers and potential for inefficiency and underreporting.[5] In a study by Rutegard and coworkers,[23] for example, anastomotic leakage after resection for rectal cancer was underreported in the Swedish Colorectal Cancer Registry. This clearly could lead to poor quality control and potential harm to patients.

One study revealed that companies, such as Merck, Glaxo, SmithKline, and Sanofi-Aventis, routinely published negative results and there were no statistical differences observed over the study duration.[12] This bolsters the argument that trial sponsors are indeed reporting disappointing outcomes. However, despite the positive impressions garnered by this study, Thayer[24] revealed that Merck and Schering-Plough faced a major backlash for withholding negative clinical results to continue profiting from their blockbuster cholesterol-lowering drugs. Although this is an older study it makes the point that the pharmaceutical industry often puts profits before safety. Additionally, Hwang and Ben-Jacob[16] analyzed the impact of public announcements regarding positive versus negative trial results. They concluded that stock performance was negatively impacted by negative trial outcomes and persisted for an extended period of time. Clearly this could affect a company's decision to release discouraging results. Clearly, profits should not be placed above the safety of patients.

RECOMMENDATIONS AND A CALL TO ACTION

Based on the evidence, a call to action is required to reverse this paradigm. The following recommendations could be helpful in beginning this dialogue:

Recommendation 1: When available, the data from well-designed trials could easily be posted immediately on ClinicalTrials.gov,[13] European Union's Clinical Trials Directive,[14] and the World Health Organization's International Trials Registry Platform.[15] Researchers have a responsibility to patients and the scientific community to publish this information. The sharing of data should be mandatory.[9,25]

Recommendation 2: Submission of a well written and statistically accurate article to a high-impact peer-reviewed journal remains essential. It is clear that negative results are notoriously underreported or altered.[20]

Recommendation 3: Researchers have a social and ethical obligation to inform the public and the medical community at large regarding trial conclusions.[26,27] Therefore, it is suggested that protocols be established to ensure that future trials are registered and published within a reasonable period of time irrespective of outcomes. This should be facilitated through the use of protocol templates, which could also aid in more expedient institutional review board reviews.[28]

Recommendation 4: The collective research community should aid in the formation of a pharma consortium to create guidelines facilitating the publication of negative results unimpeded by reviewer bias. This requires that reviewers undergo training on appropriate handling of articles that are submitted garnering less than favorable results. Reviewers must be vigilant in fairly evaluating these articles.[21]

SUMMARY

Researchers must stand with the industry giants and publish negative data post haste. Anything less seems irresponsible and could lead to wasted resources, time, and additional trials by unwitting parties for therapies that do not work.

Publishing negative outcomes could have a positive effect on patients. The quintessential example involved the COURAGE trial, which proved that cardiovascular stenting was no more effective than medical treatment in certain conditions. As with other similar scenarios, this resulted in a therapeutic sea change that forestalled thousands of unnecessary operations and altered the standard of care while saving millions of dollars in unfounded medical interventions.

The bottom line is that publishing negative results advances science while protecting patients and must be facilitated. Although this may present some challenges, researchers and sponsors must stay the course while protecting the public and other sponsors from inextricable harm. In not doing so, the death of patients may ensue because of time wasted on unproven therapies. In our world "time is tissue."

DISCLOSURE

The author has nothing to disclose.

REFERENCES

1. Brassington I. The ethics of reporting all the results of clinical trials. Br Med Bull 2017;121(1):19–29.
2. Brown A. Understanding pharmaceutical research manipulation in the context of accounting manipulation. J Law Med Ethics 2013;41(3):611–9.
3. Aronowitz R. Screen for prostate cancer in New York's skid row: history and implications. Am J Public Health 2014;104:70–6.
4. Beauchamp TL, Saghai Y. The historical foundations of the research-practice distinction in bioethics. Theor Med Bioeth 2012;33(1):45–56.
5. Song SY, Koo DH, Jung SY, et al. The significance of the trial outcome was associated with publication rate and time to publication. J Clin Epidemiol 2017;84:78–84.
6. Ovosi JO, Ibrahim MS, Bello-Ovosi BO. Randomized controlled trials: Ethical and scientific issues in the choice of placebo or active control. Ann Afr Med 2017;16(3):97–100.
7. National Commission for the Protection of Human Subjects of Biomedical and Behvioral Research. Belmont Report. US Department of Health & Human Services. Office for Human Research Protections. HHS.gov; 1978.
8. World Medical Association. World Medical Association Declaration of Helsinki ethical principles for medical research involving human subjects. JAMA 2013;310(20):2191–4.
9. Pisani E, AbouZahr A. Sharing health data: good intentions are not enough. Bull World Health Organ 2010;88:462–6.
10. Nygaard I. The importance of publishing trials with negative results [Editorial]. Am J Obstet Gynecol 2017;216. doi:10. 1016.ajog.2017.03.014
11. Unger JM, Barlow WE, Ramsey SD, et al. The scientific impact of positive and negative phase 3 cancer clinical trials. JAMA Oncol 2016;2(7):875–81.
12. Jimenez-Cotes EA, Mejia-Cardona L, Donado-Gomez JH. Publication trend of clinical trials with negative results funded by pharmaceutical industries for the 2007-2012 period. Revista Ciencias de la Salud 2015;13(1):55–62.
13. Califf R, Zarin D, Kramer J, et al. Characteristics of clinical trials registered in ClinicalTrials.gov, 2007-2010. JAMA 2012;307(17):1838–47.
14. Kenter MJ, Cohen AF. Re-engineering the European Union Clinical Trials Directive. Lancet 2012;379(9828):1765–7.
15. Kannan S, Gowri S. Clinical trials in allied medical fields: A cross-sectional analysis of World Health Organization International Clinical Trial Registry Platform. J Ayurveda Integr Med 2016;7(1):48–52.
16. Hwang T, Ben-Jacob E. Stock market returns and clinical trial results of investigational compounds: an event study analysis of large biopharmaceutical companies. PLoS One 2013;8(8):e71966.
17. U.S. Food and Drug Administration/Office of Good Clinical Practice. Civil money penalties relating to the clinicaltrials.gov data bank: guidance document. 2018. Available at: https://www.fda.gov/regulatoryinformation/guidance/ucm607652.htm.
18. Goldacre B, DeVito NJ, Heneghan C, et al. Compliance with requirement to report results on the EU clinical trials register: cohort study and web resource. BMJ 2018;362:K3218.
19. Kim D, Hedgeman B. FDA seeks civil monetary penalties measures to enforce compliance with ClinicalTrials.gov requirements. Posted in Agency Information, FDA; 2018.

20. Anderson ML, Chiswell K, Peterson ED, et al. Compliance with results reporting at clinical trials.gov. N Engl J Med 2015;372:1031–9.
21. Chiavetta NM, Martins ARS, Henriques ICR, et al. Differences in methodological quality between positive and negative published clinical trials. J Adv Nurs 2014; 70(10):2389–403.
22. Howard D, Shen Y. Trends in PCI volume after negative results from the COURAGE trial. Health Serv Res 2014;49(1):153–70.
23. Rutegård M, Kverneng Hultberg D, Angenete E, et al. Substantial underreporting of anastomotic leakage after anterior resection for rectal cancer in the Swedish Colorectal Cancer Registry. Acta Oncol 2017;56(12):1741–5.
24. Thayer A. Trial results roil drug companies: pharmaceuticals Merck, Schering Plough are under fire for withholding negative clinical trial data. Chem Eng News 2008;86(14):11.
25. Taichman D, Sahni P, Pinborg A, et al. Data sharing statements for clinical trials: a requirement of the International Committee of Medical Journal Editors. JAMA 2017;317(24):2491–2.
26. Alley A, Seo J, Hong S. Reporting results of research involving human subjects: an ethical obligation. J Korean Med Sci 2015;30(6):673–5.
27. Sibanda M, Summers R, Meyer J. Publication trends of clinical trials performed in South Africa. S Afr Med J 2016;106(5):61.
28. Hudson K, Lauer M, Collins F. Toward a new era of trust and transparency in clinical trials. J Am Med Assoc 2016;316(13):1353–4.

IX. Western University College of Podiatric Medicine

IX. Western University College of
Podiatric Medicine

Development and Evaluation of a Surgical Direct Assessment Tool for Resident Training

David Shofler, DPM, MSHS*, Steven Cooperman, BS,
Emily Shibata, BS, Eric Duffin, BS, Jarrod Shapiro, DPM

KEYWORDS

- Competency • Surgery • Assessment • Podiatric medicine • Training • Education

KEY POINTS

- There is precedence for direct assessment tools within many surgical fields that have been validated for evaluation of resident performance; this study considers application to the evaluation of residents of podiatric medicine and surgery.
- The direct assessment tool created for the evaluation of surgical competency was shown to be a reliable indicator of resident performance and may be a starting point as competency-based assessment methods in podiatric medicine and surgery are considered.
- Along with the ability for direct assessment, the tool was shown to provide the opportunity for valuable direct, case-specific feedback.

INTRODUCTION

In podiatric surgery, assessment of surgical competency is lacking. Currently, a system of minimum activity volume (MAV) numbers is used.[1] These numbers represent the fixed minimum volume of surgical cases necessary to be logged before graduation from an accredited residency program.

Although MAVs ensure that residents have a sufficient number of repetitions of categorized surgical procedures before graduation, weaknesses with this approach have been noted. First, MAVs only reference activity volume. There is no assurance that the procedures are being performed correctly or competently, or if improvement in specific areas is necessary. No feedback is generated, and no skill level is identified. Second, MAVs have been found to be ineffective and arbitrary by residency directors and

Department of Podiatric Medicine, Surgery, and Biomechanics, Western University College of Podiatric Medicine, 309 East 2nd Street, Pomona, CA 91766, USA
* Corresponding author.
E-mail address: dshofler@westernu.edu

Clin Podiatr Med Surg 37 (2020) 391–400
https://doi.org/10.1016/j.cpm.2019.12.014
0891-8422/20/© 2019 Elsevier Inc. All rights reserved.

podiatric.theclinics.com

podiatric surgery residents. A 2015 investigation published in the *Journal of Foot and Ankle Surgery* surveyed podiatric surgery residency directors and residents nationwide.[2] Respondents identified all of the existing MAV procedural requirements as being too low in number. Furthermore, the consensus opinion of directors and residents was that the use of MAVs was ineffective, and that a method involving direct assessment would have the potential to be more effective.

Methods of direct assessment are becoming more integral in surgical training across an array of surgical specialties and subspecialties.[3,4] Nonetheless, standardized methods of direct assessment are not commonly used in the training of podiatric medicine and surgery residents.

The purpose of this study was to create and assess a standardized direct assessment form to be used in the training of residents of podiatric medicine and surgery. The hypothesis of the authors was that the use of a standardized, competency-based, direct surgical assessment may be an effective tool to aid in resident training.

MATERIALS/METHODS
Assessment Tool Creation

The study was performed in two stages. In the first stage, a standardized, competency-based direct surgical assessment form was created. A medical literature review was initially performed; including a review of the surgical training literature across specialty and subspecialty training.[4–13] The initial tool incorporated a total of eight elements in a single two-sided page direct assessment form. Feedback was solicited from 14 podiatric practitioners involved in residency training, and following a series of revisions, the final version of the form was developed. The final version of the assessment tool evaluated eight different elements of surgical proficiency: (1) general respect for tissue, (2) instrument handling, (3) knowledge of the procedure, (4) use of assistants, (5) flow of operation and forward planning, (6) knowledge of instruments, (7) time and motion, and (8) overall performance (**Fig. 1**). These eight elements were evaluated in terms of level of proficiency on a five-point scale, ranging from 1 (basic knowledge) to 5 (expert) in each of the eight categories. An open response section at the bottom of the scoring system allowed for free feedback from the surgeon completing the form. Detailed scoring explanations were included on the opposite side of the form (**Fig. 2**).

Evaluation Using the Assessment Tool

After obtaining written consent to participate in the study, the form was distributed to six residents of a single podiatric medicine and surgery residency program, two for each of 3 residency years. Residents asked attending physicians to complete the forms immediately following surgical cases. Forms were collected and reliability assessment was performed. Intraclass correlation coefficients were generated for each of the numerical response items, and a summary of the results incorporated the relative reliability of each of the numerical response items. Residents were also asked to provide feedback about their experience with the assessment tool.

RESULTS

Using the resident surgical assessment tool, six podiatric surgery residents from a single residency program of podiatric medicine and surgery were evaluated. The residents represented 3 different years of training, with two evaluated from each year. There were 121 completed direct assessment forms, completed by 16 attending physicians (**Fig. 3, Table 1**). There were a total of 58, 30, and 33 forms completed

Name: _____   Postgraduate yr of training: 1 2 3
Assessor: _____
Procedure: _____
Date: _____

Please rate the resident's performance using the following scale.

General respect for tissue	Basic Knowledge 1	Novice 2	Intermediate 3	Advanced 4	Expert 5	
	often used unnecessary force on tissue or caused damage via inappropriate use of instruments		Handled tissue carefully but on occasion caused inadvertent damaged		Dependably handled tissue, caused minimal damage	N/A
Instrument handling	1 Repeatedly makes tentative or awkward moves with instruments	2	3 Competent use of instruments although occasionally appeared stiff or awkward	4	5 Fluid moves with instruments and no awkwardness	N/A
Knowledge of the procedure	Basic knowledge. needed instruction during most operative steps.	2	3 Knew all important aspects of the operation	4	5 Obviously familiar with the entire procedure including small details	N/A
Use of assistants	1 Consistently placed assistants poorly or didn't use assistants	2	3 Used assistants appropriately most of the time	4	5 Strategically used assistants at all times	N/A
Flow of operation and forward planning	1 Frequently stopped operating or needed to discuss next move	2	3 Demonstrated ability for forward planning with steady progression of procedure	4	5 Obviously planned course of operation with effortless flow from one move to the next	N/A
Knowledge of instruments	1 Frequently asked for the wrong instrument or used an inappropriate instrument	2	3 Knew the names of most instruments and used appropriate instrument for the task	4	5 Obviously familiar with the required instruments and their names	N/A
Time and Motion	1 Many unnecessary moves	2	3 Efficient time/motion but some unnecessary moves	4	5 Every movement functional, maximal efficiency	N/A

	Basic Knowledge	Novice	Intermediate	Advanced	Expert
Overall Performance	1 Below expectations	2	3 Neutral	4	5 Meets or exceeds expectations

Feedback:

_____
_____
_____

Fig. 1. The podiatry surgery resident assessment form. The form provides for assessment of overall performance and for 8 individual items: general respect for tissue, instrument handling, knowledge of the procedure, use of assistants, flow of operation and forward planning, knowledge of instruments, time and motion, and overall performance.

for post-graduate years 1, 2, and 3, respectively. Strong, statistically significant, positive correlations were evident between resident year and score across each of the eight assessment items, and with overall resident performance ($r = 0.995$; $P = .001$). The mean score across the eight items was the highest for third-year residents with 4.40, followed by second-year residents with 3.84, and finally first-year residents with 3.05. The lowest mean scoring items were "flow of operation and forward planning" and "time and motion" for first-year residents, "use of assistants" for second-year residents, and "general respect for tissue" for third-year residents. The highest scoring item was "knowledge of instruments" among first-year

Please read through the NIH Competency Proficiency Scale as well as each section of the survey before attempting to assess a surgical procedure.

Competencies Proficiency Scale

The NIH Proficiency Scale is an instrument used to measure one's ability to demonstrate a competency on the job. The scale captures a wide range of ability levels and organizes them into five steps; from "Fundamental Awareness" to "Expert".

In combination with the Proficiency Map for a specific occupation, an individual can compare their current level of proficiency to top performers in the same occupation. This scale serves as the guide to understanding the expected proficiency level of top performers at each grade level.

Score	Proficiency Level	Description
N/A	*Not Applicable*	You are not required to apply or demonstrate this competency. This competency is not applicable to your position.
1	*Fundamental Awareness* (basic knowledge)	You have a common knowledge or an understanding of basic techniques and concepts. • Focus is on learning.
2	*Novice* (limited experience)	You have the level of experience gained in a classroom and/or experimental scenarios or as a trainee on-the-job. You are expected to need help when performing this skill. • Focus is on developing through on-the-job experience; • You understand and can discuss terminology, concepts, principles, and issues related to this competency; • You utilize the full range of reference and resource materials in this competency.
3	*Intermediate* (practical application)	You are able to successfully complete tasks in this competency as requested. Help from an expert may be required from time to time, but you can usually perform the skill independently. • Focus is on applying and enhancing knowledge or skill; • You have applied this competency to situations occasionally while needing minimal guidance to perform successfully; • You understand and can discuss the application and implications of changes to processes, policies, and procedures in this area.
4	*Advanced* (applied theory)	You can perform the actions associated with this skill without assistance. You are certainly recognized within your immediate organization as "a person to ask" when difficult questions arise regarding this skill. • Focus is on broad organizational/professional issues; • You have consistently provided practical/relevant ideas and perspectives on process or practice improvements which may easily be implemented; • You are capable of coaching others in the application of this competency by translating complex nuances relating to this competency into easy to understand terms; • You participate in senior level discussions regarding this competency; • You assist in the development of reference and resource materials in this competency.
5	*Expert* (recognized authority)	You are known as an expert in this area. You can provide guidance, troubleshoot and answer questions related to this area of expertise and the field where the skill is used. • Focus is strategic; • You have demonstrated consistent excellence in applying this competency across multiple projects and/or organizations; • You are considered the "go to" person in this area within NIH and/or outside organizations; • You create new applications for and/or lead the development of reference and resource materials for this competency; • You are able to diagram or explain the relevant process elements and issues in relation to organizational issues and trends in sufficient detail during discussions and presentations, to foster a greater understanding among internal and external colleagues and constituents.

Note: The NIH Proficiency Scale was updated to facilitate the migration to the HHS Learning Management System. (Updated January 12, 2009)

The term "Failed to" in the survey does not suggest that an action was not performed but instead suggests that the attending physician was required to remind or step in for the resident.

Fig. 2. The reverse side of the podiatry surgery resident assessment form. The form provides detailed descriptions of the different levels of assessment, ranging from: "Fundamental/Awareness (Basic Knowledge)" as a score of 1, to "Expert (Recognized Authority)" as a score of 5. (*Adapted from* National Institutes of Health. Office of Human Resources. Competencies Proficiency Scale. Available at: https://hr.nih.gov/working-nih/competencies/competencies-proficiency-scale.)

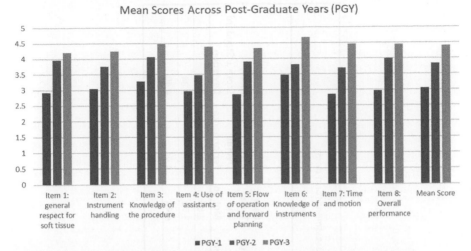

Fig. 3. Mean scores among post-graduate years in corresponding assessment items.

residents, "knowledge of the procedure" among second-year residents, and "knowledge of instruments" among third-year residents. Across attending physicians, the intraclass correlation was 0.84 for overall resident performance score.

Feedback from residents was encouraging overall, with residents noting that the forms helped start a dialogue with attending physicians following surgical cases. The most common suggestion by residents was for additional space on the assessment form for attending physician comments, including space for each individual assessment item.

DISCUSSION

The results of this study reflect the potential utility of standardized assessment in podiatric surgical training. In general, resident assessment is a critical component of surgical training, and largely serves two purposes. First, assessment is formative: it can provide feedback for surgical residents, thereby stimulating improvement and reinforcing learning. Second, assessment is summative, serving to identify resident skill level and competence.[13] The use of the created forms aided both purposes. The forms were readily completed by attending physicians, provided value to current residents, and helped assess procedural competence.

Martin and Reznick[5] and the Surgical Education Research Group at the University of Toronto created an Objective Structured Assessment of Technical Skill (OSATS) tool in 1994 to objectively assess technical skill during an operation.[6] The OSATS testing was based on a format consistent with the typical Objective Structured Clinical Examination, in which each examinee performed several clinical tasks at different stations and was accompanied with a global rating form that included seven elements, which were graded on a five-point Likert-type scale. In the original evaluation of this tool, Martin and colleagues evaluated 20 surgical residents using the OSATS tool during a six-station live animal model examination and a bench model examination. There were found to be no significant differences between the two models, and increasing competence was noted with increasing years of surgical residency.

In a follow-up study of the OSATS tool in 1997, Reznick and colleagues[7] evaluated 48 general surgery residents to determine the reliability of an eight-station, 2-hour OSATS examination. In this study, the global rating form used to assess technical skill

Table 1
Number of forms completed and mean scores among post-graduate resident years for corresponding assessment form items

Post-graduate Year	Number of Forms	Item 1: General Respect for Tissue	Item 2: Instrument Handling	Item 3: Knowledge of the Procedure	Item 4: Use of Assistants	Item 5: Flow of Operation and Forward Planning	Item 6: Knowledge of Instruments	Item 7: Time and Motion	Item 8: Overall Performance	Mean Score ± Standard Deviation
						Mean Scores				
1	58	2.93	3.05	3.29	2.96	2.85	3.47	2.85	2.97	3.05
2	30	3.97	3.77	4.07	3.48	3.90	3.80	3.70	4.00	3.84
3	33	4.21	4.24	4.48	4.38	4.33	4.67	4.45	4.44	4.40
All	121	—	—	—	—	—	—	—	$r = 0.995$	P value $= .001$

during the OSATS examination was shown to be a reliable tool for assessing surgical competency. As a result of their findings, the authors adopted the use of annual testing of technical competence within their surgical training program. Identical and modified versions of the Likert scale assessment form originally described have been validated extensively and integrated into many residency programs.[8–10] In fact, this type of form is so popular, that in a 2015 systematic review by Szasz and colleagues[4] assessing the methods by which technical competence is determined in surgical trainees, Likert scales were the most common method of assessment being used.

Following the creation and success of the OSATS tool, other authors began creating, publishing, and refining their own similar version of this evaluation tool, but with unique changes to enhance the form. In 2012, to evaluate not only a resident's technical skills, but also their competency in completing an entire surgical procedure, Gofton and colleagues[11] created the Ottawa Surgical Competency Operating Room Evaluation (O-SCORE).[12] This validated tool is a nine-item scoring device, with the ninth element making this tool unique: this item is scored as a yes/no response to "Resident is able to safely perform this procedure independently," which prevents the tool from differentiating the rating based on the evaluators' perceptions of the trainee's current level of experience, but evaluates whether or not the surgery could have been completed without the attending physician present.

Hadley and colleagues[14] created another validated, novel form based off of the OSATS tool in 2015 for the evaluation resident's operative skills in pediatric neurosurgery. This form was unique in that the residents themselves were required to evaluate their own performance. In 2017, Isupov and colleagues[15] created a pilot form for assessing procedural competency among radiology residents. Isupov's newly created RAD-Score tool differed slightly from the OSATS and O-SCORE tools, in that the primary outcome measure in their study was not whether the attending physician believed that the procedure could be performed without them, but whether or not the resident felt prepared to perform procedures independently.

One of the benefits of standardized assessment is that it provides immediate feedback for residents. Feedback has been shown to be necessary and inadequate in graduate medical education.[15,16] In previous studies from various surgical fields, feedback has been shown to be a valuable teaching technique, especially in the operating room.[17–19] In podiatric medicine, direct feedback immediately after surgery has been identified by residents as the single most valuable learning resource.[2] However, feedback is often limited because of many factors: the delivery of feedback, the resident/attending relationship, and the amount of time available for feedback. Although the primary purpose of feedback is to encourage improvement in performance, there is also often a discrepancy between the attending physician providing feedback and the resident physician receiving feedback in terms of how each act is perceived.[20]

An internal survey by the department of orthopedic surgery at the Carolinas Medical Center found that 63% of residents were not satisfied with their feedback on operative performance, with residents most frequently citing a lack of case-specific feedback and the infrequency of feedback as a source of dissatisfaction.[21] It has been suggested that feedback is enhanced when specific examples of strengths and weaknesses are provided, especially in the setting of standardized documentation.[22–24] Additionally, in a study by Albano and colleagues,[25] 22.5% of residents viewed feedback as a stressful or intimidating event, although 97.5% in the study were shown to have a change in behavior or practice based on the feedback given.

With the creation of the current assessment tool, the most frequent comment was that the form provided residents the opportunity for open dialogue with the attending physician. At first, several of the residents noted that the evaluation form felt "awkward" and did not like the idea of "inconveniencing" their attending physicians. However, these same residents noted that they were provided quality feedback as a direct result of the tool.

When implementing a required evaluation tool, however, certain considerations apply. This includes how to ensure compliance of resident and attending physicians. Lack of compliance of residents and attending physicians can act as a barrier to implementation. This is caused by the frequency of feedback and the format of feedback. If residents and attending physicians are to complete an individual form for every surgery performed, there is increased risk of evaluation fatigue leading to evaluations that are incomplete, delinquent, or inaccurate.[26]

The effect of negative feedback on junior residents should also be a consideration. Although it is expected that junior residents receive lower scores than senior residents, lower scores can affect the willingness of junior residents to continually seek feedback.[27] In a study by Ode and colleagues[20] implementing a similar evaluation tool to assess orthopedic surgical skills competency, it was shown that survey compliance increased with increasing post-graduate year.

There are several limitations of this study. First, this study was conducted at a single residency program over a 3-month period. An expanded, formalized pilot, conducted over the entirety of a residency year and across a representative selection of residency programs, could provide superior justification for the use of the proposed standardized assessment form. Second, analysis was not conducted regarding procedure type. Senior residents may have performed more complicated procedures, distorting the comparison between residency years. Considering the value of this instrument when applied to simple versus complex surgical procedures may be appropriate for any future investigation. Lastly, attending physicians in the present study were not blinded to the level of the resident, which may have led to confounding of the data. Future investigations could involve blinded video recordings of residents performing procedures, with evaluations of the same video conducted by several different attending physicians.

SUMMARY

Although MAV requirements have value, competency-based assessment may be a helpful addition to residency training. The direct assessment form created through this study may be a starting point as competency-based assessment methods in podiatric medicine and surgery are considered.

DISCLOSURE

The authors have nothing to disclose.

REFERENCES

1. Standards and requirements for approval of podiatric medicine and surgery residents. Council of Podiatric Medical Education web site; 2015. Available at: https://www.cpme.org/files/CPME%20320%20final%20June%202015.pdf. Accessed September 14, 2019.
2. Shofler D, Chuang T, Argade N. The residency training experience in podiatric medicine and surgery. J Foot Ankle Surg 2015;54(4):607–14.
3. Jeray KJ, Frick SL. A survey of resident perspectives on surgical case minimums and the impact on milestones, graduation, credentialing, and preparation for practice: AOA critical issues. J Bone Joint Surg Am 2014;96(23):e195.

4. Szasz P, Louridas M, Harris KA, et al. Assessing technical competence in surgical trainees: a systematic review. Ann Surg 2015;261(6):1046–55.
5. Martin JA, Reznick RK. Reliability and validity of an instrument to evaluate operative skill in surgical residents. Can J Surg 1994;37:342.
6. Martin JA, Regehr G, Reznick R, et al. Objective structured assessment of technical skill (OSATS) for surgical residents. Br J Surg 1997;84(2):273–8.
7. Reznick R, Regehr G, MacRae H, et al. Testing technical skill via an innovative "bench station" examination. Am J Surg 1997;173(3):226–30.
8. Hance J, Aggarwal R, Stanbridge R, et al. Objective assessment of technical skills in cardiac surgery. Eur J Cardiothorac Surg 2005;28(1):157–62.
9. Vassiliou MC, Feldman LS, Andrew CG, et al. A global assessment tool for evaluation of intraoperative laparoscopic skills. Am J Surg 2005;190(1):107–13.
10. Chipman JG, Schmitz CC. Using objective structured assessment of technical skills to evaluate a basic skills simulation curriculum for first-year surgical residents. J Am Coll Surg 2009;209:364–70.e2.
11. Gofton W, Dudek N, Wood T, et al. The Ottawa Surgical Competency Operating Room Evaluation (O-SCORE): a tool to assess surgical competence. Acad Med 2012;87:1401–7.
12. MacEwan MJ, Dudek NL, Wood TJ, et al. Continued validation of the O-SCORE (Ottawa Surgical Competency Operating Room Evaluation): use in the simulated environment. Teach Learn Med 2016;28(1):72–9.
13. Dougherty P, Kasten SJ, Reynolds RK, et al. Intraoperative assessment of residents. J Grad Med Educ 2013;5(2):333–4.
14. Hadley C, Lam SK, Briceño V, et al. Use of a formal assessment instrument for evaluation of resident operative skills in pediatric neurosurgery. J Neurosurg Pediatr 2015;16(5):497–504.
15. Isupov I, McInnes MD, Hamstra SJ, et al. Development of RAD-score: a tool to assess the procedural competence of diagnostic radiology residents. AJR Am J Roentgenol 2017;208(4):820–6.
16. Jensen AR, Wright AS, Kim S, et al. Educational feedback in the operating room: a gap between resident and faculty perceptions. Am J Surg 2012;204:248–55.
17. Cox SS1, Swanson MS. Identification of teaching excellence in operating room and clinic settings. Am J Surg 2002;183(3):251–5.
18. Dath D, Hoogenes J, Matsumoto ED, et al. Exploring how surgeon teachers motivate residents in the operating room. Am J Surg 2013;205(2):151–5.
19. Roberts NK, Brenner MJ, Williams RG, et al. Capturing the teachable moment: a grounded theory study of verbal teaching interactions in the operating room. Surgery 2012;151(5):643–50.
20. Ode GE, Buck JS, Wally M, et al. Obstacles affecting the implementation of the O-SCORE for assessment of orthopedic surgical skills competency. J Surg Educ 2019;76(3):881–92.
21. Laughlin T, Brennan A, Brailovsky C. Effect of field notes on confidence and perceived competence: survey of faculty and residents. Can Fam Physician 2012;58(6):e352–6.
22. Vollmer CM Jr, Newman LR, Huang G, et al. Perspectives on intraoperative teaching: divergence and convergence between learner and teacher. J Surg Educ 2011;68(6):485–94.
23. Sender Liberman A, Liberman M, Steinert Y, et al. Surgery residents and attending surgeons have different perceptions of feedback. Med Teach 2005; 27(5):470–2.

24. Reddy ST, Zegarek MH, Fromme HB, et al. Barriers and facilitators to effective feedback: a qualitative analysis of data from multispecialty resident focus groups. J Grad Med Educ 2015;7(2):214–9.
25. Albano S, Quadri SA, Farooqui M, et al. Resident perspective on feedback and barriers for use as an educational tool. Cureus 2019;11(5):e4633.
26. Shah N, Thompson B, Averill P, et al. Increasing the rate of return of resident rotation evaluations by their attending physicians in an in-patient psychiatric facility. Acad Psychiatry 2007;31(6):439–42.
27. Kannappan A, Yip DT, Lodhia NA, et al. The effect of positive and negative verbal feedback on surgical skills performance and motivation. J Surg Educ 2012;69(6): 798–801.

Efficacy and Safety of Efinaconazole 10% Solution in the Treatment of Onychomycosis in Diabetic Patients

David Shofler, DPM, MSHS*, Elnaz Hamedani, BA, BS,
Jonathan Seun, BS, Ricardo Navarrete, BA, BS, Rohan Thamby, MS,
Lawrence Harkless, DPM

KEYWORDS

- Onychomycosis • Diabetes • Efinaconazole • Topical • Antifungal

KEY POINTS

- Diabetic patients are more likely to suffer from onychomycosis and may be more likely to suffer from complications due to the condition.
- In the present study, the clinical efficacy of efinaconazole 10% topical solution was not found to correlate with glycemic control.
- Efinaconazole 10% topical solution may represent a useful option in treating diabetic patients with onychomycosis, including those with extensive fungal involvement of the nail plate.

INTRODUCTION

Onychomycosis, a common pathology of the toenails, is especially prevalent among diabetic patients. Although an estimated 30.3 million Americans suffer from diabetes, nearly one-third of diabetics have been found to have toenail onychomycosis.[1,2] Diabetics have been found to be 2.77 times more likely than nondiabetics to suffer from the condition.[2]

The presence of onychomycosis is of heightened concern among diabetics. Diabetic patients with onychomycosis have been found to suffer a 3-fold higher incidence of gangrene and/or foot ulcer than diabetic patients without onychomycosis.[3] Diabetic patients with onychomycosis have also been shown to suffer increased risk of bacterial infections, including cellulitis, and the condition can directly lead to pain, discomfort, and decreased quality of life.[4,5]

Efinaconazole 10% solution is a relatively new triazole antifungal agent, developed specifically for the topical treatment of onychomycosis.[6] The solution was developed

Department of Podiatric Medicine, Surgery, and Biomechanics, Western University College of Podiatric Medicine, 309 E 2nd Street, Pomona, CA 91766, USA
* Corresponding author.
E-mail address: dshofler@westernu.edu

Clin Podiatr Med Surg 37 (2020) 401–407
https://doi.org/10.1016/j.cpm.2019.12.015   podiatric.theclinics.com

with consideration of the existing triazole antifungals, itraconazole and fluconazole, with the formulation developed to more effectively penetrate the nail plate.[7]

Although the medication has been studied in cohorts that included diabetic patients, diabetic patients have not been the specific focus of a clinical investigation evaluating the efficacy and safety of efinaconazole 10% solution. Further, previous investigations have excluded diabetic patients whom did not exhibit glycemic control or for whom more than 50% of the target toenail was clinically involved.[8]

The purpose of this study was to evaluate the efficacy and safety of efinaconazole 10% topical solution among a cohort of diabetic subjects. It was hypothesized that the medication would retain efficacy and safety among this study population. The goal was to yield information that would aid in the clinical management of diabetic patients suffering from onychomycosis.

METHODS

The objective of this noncomparative, open-label study was to determine the efficacy of topical efinaconazole 10% for toenail onychomycosis among subjects with diabetes mellitus. Specific indicators to measure efficacy of treatment were the complete cure rate, mycological cure rate, and treatment success rate. Complete cure rate was designated as the primary efficacy endpoint. Safety was evaluated by the incidence and nature of treatment-associated adverse events, which were recorded at each follow-up visit.

Complete cure was defined as 0% clinical involvement and mycological cure. Clinical cure was defined as 0% clinical involvement of the target toenail. Treatment success was defined as less than or equal to 10% clinical involvement of the target toenail. Mycological cure was defined as negative positive potassium hydroxide (KOH) examination and negative fungal culture of the target toenail sample.

The primary efficacy endpoint was the proportion of subjects achieving complete cure at week 50. The secondary efficacy endpoints included mycological cure rate, treatment success rate, and clinical cure rate. Safety endpoints included the type and frequency of adverse events. Intended enrollment was 40 subjects.

Pearson correlations were calculated between hemoglobin A1C values and the 3 efficacy endpoints: complete cure rate, mycological cure rate, and treatment success rate. These correlations were performed using the Statistical Package for Social Sciences Version 25, and statistical significance was set as $P<.05$.

SUBJECT ELIGIBILITY

Subject eligibility was determined by inclusion and exclusion criteria. To be considered for inclusion, a positive KOH wet mount was required, combined with a fungal culture positive for either trichophyton rubrum or trichophyton mentagrophytes. Involvement of minimum 20% of the target great toenail was required for inclusion. A negative pregnancy screen was required among women of child-bearing age. These women were required to be on oral contraceptive throughout the study duration. Subjects were excluded if any of the following exclusion criteria were met:

- Diagnosis of a nondermatophyte fungus infection, diagnosis of superficial white onychomycosis
- Diagnosis of peripheral arterial disease or anatomic abnormalities of the target toenail
- Inability to follow through with all requisite office visits
- Routine use of a systemic corticosteroid, routine use of a systemic immunomodulator, or history of systemic antifungals within the prior 5 years.

- Active interdigital tinea pedis refractory to topical antifungal treatments
- Known hypersensitivity to efinaconazole
- Use, within the month preceding screening, of topical antifungal agents, topical antiinflammatory agents to the toes
- Any history of oral systemic antifungal with known activity against dermatophytes

A signed written informed consent was required before subject enrollment. Local institutional review board approval was obtained before study commencement.

SUBJECT ASSESSMENT

Eligible subjects were dispensed efinaconazole 10% topical solution, as well as instructions on how to appropriately apply the solution to the target great toenail. If more toenails were affected, subjects were instructed on how to appropriately apply the solution to all of the affected toenails. Subjects were assessed at enrollment and at every 10 weeks until week 50 (at weeks 10, 20, 30, 40, and 50). At each patient visit, assessment of the target great toenail was conducted using digital planimetry. Following planimetry imaging, toenails were debrided at each visit. A final KOH wet mount and fungal culture were ordered at the subject's final visit at week 50. Subjects were considered to have completed the study after attending the week 50 follow-up evaluation.

RESULTS

A total of 40 diabetic subjects were enrolled at a single investigational site, a hospital-based outpatient podiatric clinic (**Fig. 1**). The average age of enrolled subjects was 58.15 ± 9.71 years (**Table 1**). The average hemoglobin A1C of enrolled subjects was 7.71% +/− 1.68%. Of the 40 enrolled subjects, 19 (47.50%) identified using injectable insulin and 27 (67.50%) identified using oral hypoglycemics at the time of enrollment. A total of 4 subjects (10.00%) were on dialysis at the time of enrollment. Most of the enrolled subjects were Hispanic (31 of 40, 77.50%); there were 4 African-American subjects (10.00%), 4 White subjects (10.00%), and 1 Asian subject (2.50%).

A total of 36 of 40 subjects reached week 50 and completed the study (90.00%). The 4 subjects (10.00%) who did not complete the study were lost to follow-up. On a per protocol basis, the average nail involvement at enrollment was 56.01% +/− 22.38%. The range of nail involvement was 20.40% to 92.70%.

SUBJECT OUTCOMES

Complete cure, defined as 0% clinical involvement combined with mycological cure, was achieved in 4 of the 36 subjects (11.11%) who completed the study. The same 4, and no additional, subjects obtained clinical cure, defined as 0% clinical involvement. A total of 8 subjects (20%) achieved either clinical cure or treatment success, which was defined as less than or equal to 10% clinical involvement. Mycological cure, defined as negative KOH examination and negative fungal culture of the target toenail sample, was achieved in 21 of the 36 subjects (58.33%). The average clinical involvement of the target toenail at week 50 was 31.75% +/− 25.58%.

Of the 36 subjects completing the study, 19 (52.78%) exhibited clinical involvement of greater than 50% of the target toenail. Considering these subjects separately, average nail involvement at enrollment was 73.85% (+/− 13.97%), and at study completion the average nail involvement was 44.90% (+/− 26.72%). Of these 19 subjects, one subject (5.26%) achieved complete cure, 2 subjects achieved either

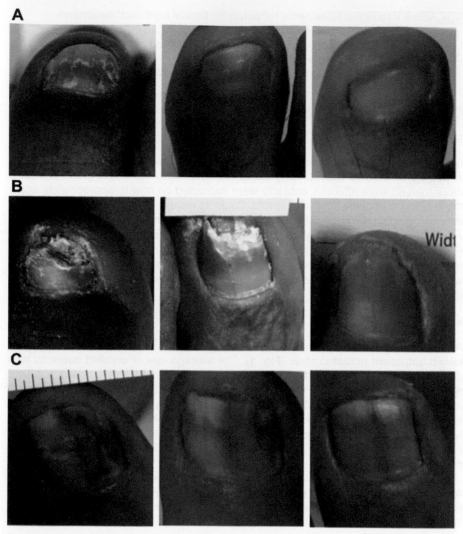

Fig. 1. Representative photographs of three subjects exhibiting improvement in the clinical involvement of the target toenail over the duration of the study. Photographs are of three subjects (A–C) at enrollment, 20-week follow-up visits, and 50-week follow-up visits respectively.

complete cure or treatment success (10.53%), and 7 subjects (36.84%) achieved either mycological cure or complete cure.

The remaining 17 (47.22%) exhibited less than 50% clinical involvement of the target toenail at enrollment. Of these 17 subjects, the average nail involvement at enrollment was 36.06% (+/− 8.72%), and at study completion the average nail involvement was 17.05% (+/− 13.89%). Three of the 17 (17.65%) achieved complete cure, 6 (35.30%) achieved either treatment success or complete cure, and 14 (82.35%) achieved mycological cure or complete cure.

There were a total of 4 local adverse events. There were 2 cases (5.56%) of vesicles appearing on the target toenail, 1 case (2.78%) of cellulitis limited to the leg of the

Table 1
Demographic characteristics of the study population at enrollment

Characteristics	Value
Sex No.(%)	
M	23 (57.5)
F	17 (42.5)
Age (y)	
Mean ± SD	58.15 ± 9.70
Range	33–78
Ethnicity No.(%)	
Hispanic	31(77.5)
African-American	4(10.0)
White	4(10.0)
Asian	1(2.5)
Insulin Use No.(%)	
Yes	19(47.5)
No	21(52.5)
Oral Diabetes Medication No.(%)	
Yes	28(70.0)
No	12(30.0)
Neuropathy No.(%)	
Yes	27(67.5)
No	13(32.5)
Dialysis No.(%)	
Yes	4(10.0)
No	36(90.0)
HbA1C	
Mean ± SD	7.71 ± 1.68

same lower extremity as the target toenail, and 1 case (2.78%) of a new-onset verruca of the same lower extremity as the target toenail.

There were no notable associations between hemoglobin A1C level and efficacy endpoints. For complete cure rate, the correlation coefficient was 0.019; for mycological cure rate, the correlation coefficient was 0.135; for treatment success, the correlation coefficient was 0.017. None of these 3 correlations reached statistical significance.

DISCUSSION

In the present study, efinaconazole 10% solution was found to be safe and efficacious among a cohort of diabetic patients not restricted by either glycemic control or amount of nail involvement. Efficacy outcomes were not found to be associated with level of glycemic control. Although subjects with less than 50% clinical involvement of the target toenail at enrollment exhibited superior efficacy outcomes compared with those with greater than 50% clinical involvement of the target toenail, the latter group exhibited a larger reduction in the percentage of clinical involvement of the target toenail.

The results of this study reflect comparably with previous investigations. On a per protocol basis, the primary efficacy endpoint, complete cure rate at week 50, was achieved in 11.11% of subjects. As reference, 2 large multicenter controlled clinical trials achieved complete cure rates of 17.8% and 15.2%, respectively.[8] Considering only the diabetic subjects from these 2 trials, the complete cure rates were 13.0% and 18.8%, respectively.[9]

Differences in enrollment criteria may account for the small difference of reported outcomes. In the present study, enrollment was not limited by clinical involvement of the target toenail; in the former studies, a maximum of 50% clinical involvement of the target toenail was permitted. Restricting our results to the subset of subjects who had less than 50% clinical involvement of the target toenail yields a complete cure rate of 17.65%, more in parallel with previous findings.

Mycological cure rates also approximate these 2 previous studies. A total of 58.33% of subjects in the present study achieved mycological cure; the rates reported in the 2 aforementioned trials were 55.2% and 53.4%, respectively. Among the diabetic patients in the cohorts of these 2 trials, the rate of mycological cure was found to be 56.5%.[9]

It should be noted that in the present study, diabetic patients were enrolled regardless of their level of glycemic control; in the former study, only diabetic patients exhibiting glycemic control were permitted. In the authors' study, the average hemoglobin A1C was 7.71%, with a standard deviation of 1.68%.

The most common adverse event, application site vesicles, occurred in 5.56% of subjects completing the study (2/36). The 2 large controlled trials identified the occurrence of this adverse event as 2.0% and 1.2%, respectively.[8] Although cellulitis of the leg and verrucae, each of which occurred in one subject, have not been previously reported as possible adverse events, neither of these cases were believed to be a likely direct consequence of the medication.

Another natural point of comparison is an earlier open-label study of ciclopirox 8% nail lacquer topical solution.[10] With the same number of subjects completing this earlier study (36), the reported complete cure rate was 4.4%. Rates of insulin and oral hypoglycemic use slightly differed between the 2 studies—33% of the subjects had used injectable insulin and 82% of the subjects had used oral hypoglycemics in the prior study—whereas in the present study, 47.50% of subjects identified using injectable insulin and 67.50% of subjects identified using oral hypoglycemics at the time of enrollment.

Recent, smaller investigations of efinaconazole 10% solution have also been conducted. Bonhert and colleagues[11] suggested a possible benefit when the medication was combined with laser therapy. Canavan and colleagues[12] suggested that efinaconazole 10% solution may retain efficacy when combined with nail polish but that the combination may affect the quality of the nail polish.

Limitations of the present study include the lack of diversity among the subject population, as just more than three-quarters of subjects self-identified as Hispanic. This may limit the generalizability of these results, for example, when considering other patient populations. Relatedly, Cook-Bolden and Lin performed a cohort analysis of Latino subjects using the earlier 2 large multicenter controlled trials.[13] These investigators found that the efficacy of efinaconazole 10% solution was slightly higher among Latino patients than non-Latino subjects, a difference that was found to be statistically significant.

An additional limitation was the lack of a control group. As an open-label study, there was not a comparison group to confirm the findings regarding efficacy and safety. Although the results were compatible with previous studies, a future randomized, controlled study may be of value.

A final limitation concerns the assessment of toenail improvement. Although KOH wet mounts and fungal cultures are frequently used in formal investigations of onychomycosis, in practice other methods are also common and have specific advantages. Furthermore, a trend toward emphasizing patient-centered outcomes may lead to further considerations when designing investigations of onychomycosis improvement.

SUMMARY

Efinaconazole 10% solution seems to maintain efficacy and safety in the treatment of onychomycosis among diabetic patients. A follow-up randomized, controlled investigation may be helpful in supporting the findings of this study.

ACKNOWLEDGMENTS

This study was supported by a research grant from Valeant Pharmaceuticals International.

DISCLOSURE

The authors have nothing to disclose.

REFERENCES

1. Centers for Disease Control and Prevention. National diabetes statistics report: estimates of diabetes and its burden in the United States. Atlanta (GA): Centers for Disease Control and Prevention; 2017.
2. Gupta AK, Konnikov N, MacDonald P, et al. Prevalence and epidemiology of toenail onychomycosis in diabetic subjects: a multicenter study. Br J Dermatol 1998;139:665-71.
3. Gupta AK, Humke S. The prevalence and management of onychomycosis in diabetic patients. Eur J Dermatol 2000;10(5):379-84.
4. LaSenna CE, Tosti A. Patient considerations in the management of toe onychomycosis - role of efinaconazole. Patient Prefer Adherence 2015;9:887-91.
5. Vanhooteghem O, Szepetiuk G, Paurobally D, et al. Chronic interdigital dermatophytic infection: a common lesion associated with potentially severe consequences. Diabetes Res Clin Pract 2011;91(1):23-5.
6. Gupta AK, Simpson FC. Efinaconazole: a new topical treatment for onychomycosis. Skin Therapy Lett 2014;19(1):1-4.
7. Tatsumi Y, Nagashima M, Shibanushi T, et al. Mechanism of action of efinaconazole, a novel triazole antifungal agent. Antimicrob Agents Chemother 2013;57(5):2405-9.
8. Elewski BE, Rich P, Pollak R, et al. Efinaconazole 10% solution in the treatment of toenail onychomycosis: two phase III multicenter, randomized, double-blind studies. J Am Acad Dermatol 2013;68(4):600-8.
9. Vlahovic TC, Joseph WS. Efinaconazole topical, 10% for the treatment of toenail onychomycosis in patients with diabetes. J Drugs Dermatol 2014;13(10):1186-90.
10. Brenner MA1, Harkless LB, Mendicino RW, et al. Ciclopirox 8% nail lacquer topical solution for the treatment of onychomycosis in subjects with diabetes: a multicenter, open-label study. J Am Podiatr Med Assoc 2007;97(3):195-202.
11. Bonhert K, Dorizas A, Sadick NS. Efficacy of combination therapy with efinaconazole 10% solution and 1064 nm Nd:YAG laser for treatment of toenail onychomycosis. J Cosmet Laser Ther 2019;21(3):179-83.
12. Canavan TN, Bevans SL, Cantrell WC, et al. Single-center, prospective, blinded study comparing the efficacy and compatibility of efinaconazole 10% solution in treating onychomycosis with and without concurrent nail polish use. Skin Appendage Disord 2018;5(1):9-12.
13. Cook-Bolden FE, Lin T. Efinaconazole solution 10% for treatment of toenail onychomycosis in Latino patients. Cutis 2017;99(4):286-9.

The Use of Virtual Reality in Podiatric Medical Education

Jonathan Labovitz, DPM[a,*], Chandler Hubbard, DPM[b,c]

KEYWORDS

- Virtual reality • Graduate medical education • Podiatric medical education • Podiatry
- Virtual operating room • Digital learning • Educational technology

KEY POINTS

- Simulation-based training provides educational opportunities that enhance acquisition of knowledge, skills, and behaviors promoting a competency-based educational system in environments promoting patient safety.
- Virtual reality simulations have demonstrated enhanced surgical skills transferable to the real-world operating room setting.
- Expansion of educational methods to include a virtual operating room specific to the needs of podiatric surgery in the clinical curriculum at Western University of Health Sciences.
- WesternU College of Podiatric Medicine anticipates the virtual operating room enhances student engagement in podiatric surgical and interprofessional team-based training to facilitate improvements in students' knowledge and skills, and ultimately impacting patient care quality and safety.

INTRODUCTION

Technological advances have changed every industry and advancements often exceed the imagination of preceding generations. Education is no exception. In fact, educational technology has transformed teaching and learning, impacting elementary and secondary schools, undergraduate education, and graduate and professional programs. More specifically, medical education has been revolutionized by the influx of technology into classrooms, and now, into the clinical realm to educate doctors and other health professionals whether they are earning their degree, entrenched in post-graduate training, or during continuing education for practicing providers.

[a] Clinical Education and Graduate Placement, Western University of Health Sciences, College of Podiatric Medicine, 309 East 2nd Street, Pomona, CA 91766, USA; [b] Western University of Health Sciences, 309 East 2nd Street, Pomona, CA 91766, USA; [c] Chino Valley Medical Center, 5451 Walnut Avenue, Chino, CA 91710, USA
* Corresponding author.
E-mail address: jlabovitz@westernu.edu

Clin Podiatr Med Surg 37 (2020) 409–420
https://doi.org/10.1016/j.cpm.2019.12.008
0891-8422/20/© 2019 Elsevier Inc. All rights reserved.

Similar to the role of technology in other industries, the expanding role of educational technology attempts to leverage these advancements to develop more efficient and improved outcomes. In medical education, educational technology serves as a method of delivering information and boosting the experience for the students.[1] However, it should ideally be used to improve processes and resources for meaningful learning activities, which secondarily aids in delivering information and improving the experience.[2]

Simulations are a type of educational technology that creates an environment to mimic real-world situations. Although simulations involve various degrees of complexity based on the situation being replicated, the success of most simulations in medical education remains debatable because there is a lack of evidence demonstrating the significant improvements in learning outcomes translate to improved clinical outcomes.[3,4]

In this review, we focus on the role of virtual reality (VR) simulations in podiatric medicine. This is one of the newest technologies to begin permeating medical education and is something being developed and tested at the Western University of Health Sciences (WesternU) College of Podiatric Medicine (CPM).

IT WORKED FOR ME, WHY CHANGE?

Medical knowledge has been expanding exponentially. Whereas the doubling time of medical knowledge was an estimated 50 years in 1950, it accelerated to 7 years in 1980, 3.5 years in 2010, and a projected 73 days by 2020.[5] In an age where medical records are electronically recorded and accessed, and diagnostic testing and imaging with treatment is available at a click of a button, the realm of medical education remains somewhat primitive. Although the current academic system has proven to produce respectable, well-qualified doctors, can advances in education produce even better physicians and surgeons? Can physicians and surgeons get equivalent training while improving patient safety?

Many of us were educated successfully without technology playing a significant role. In fact, many health care providers only recently started using various technological advancements when caring for patients. So the old adage "it worked for me so why change" is a logical question. It begs us to ask if we really need all of these technological advances to educate future physicians and health care providers. However, in light of the changes impacting health care, we see how technological advances revolutionize patient care. These advances and future advancements can positively change medical education, ultimately impacting patient safety and quality of care.

Using and developing new technologies also allows educators to adapt how we teach to the learning styles of the student. If we cannot communicate with the student in a manner that facilitates learning, we fail to educate the student. The millennial generation are "digital native" learners and have come to expect the use of technology in education, and medical education is no exception.[6] Unlike the baby boomer and generation X learners, the millennial generation was raised surrounded by continual advances in technology, in and out of the classroom. Millennials expect immediate feedback but are often unable to handle negative feedback and are thought to be visual learners. Moreover, instructional strategies often recommended for this generation include clear objectives and standards, multimedia, social media, and smartphone apps compared with generation X learners, who enjoy and are comfortable with technology, yet they desire learning via real-world activities. Meanwhile, generation Z students who have grown up with the most recent technological developments are now enrolled in graduate health professional schools (**Table 1**).

Table 1
Generational differences in communication and learning styles

	Baby Boomers	Generation X	Millennials	Generation Z
Born	1944–1964	1965–1979	1980–1994	1995–2015
Attitude toward technology	Early information technology adaptors	Digital immigrants (independent user, acquired skill, tech savvy)	Digital natives (assimilated, technology advanced)	Always connected (dependent, does not know alternatives)
Signature technology	Television	Personal computer	Tablet or smart phone	Google glass, 3-dimensional printing, AR/VR
Communication preference	Face-to-face, telephone/email if required	Cell phone Email Text messaging	Online/mobile instant message text messaging	Facetime Instant message, text messaging
Learner traits	Facilitator led, hands-on, open to new methods	Independent, self-reliant, resourceful, problem solvers, intolerant of bureaucracy, appreciate technology	Expect immediate feedback, not accustomed to negative feedback, short attention span, sheltered, visual learners, expect technology and accommodations, style > substance	
Instructional strategies	Take in information using books and handouts, easy-to-scan memos and bulleted lists that highlight important details Face-to-face or telephone call to answer questions	Direct communication Real-world assignments Case studies Incorporate technology when possible, email with opportunity for dialogue	Clear objectives and standards, communicate via text, develop self-assessment tools, group work, incorporate technology, multimedia environment, use social media, mobile phone apps, short, quick emails to keep up to date	

Abbreviation: AR, augmented reality.

The other key reason for change relates to the more global changes of the health care environment. Limited patient availability caused by fewer operating room (OR) experiences, limited exposure to infrequent and rare conditions, and shortages of clinical training sites has impacted training. Patient safety is another critical factor driving the use of simulations. It is well established that operations performed by inexperienced surgeons have poorer outcomes. Therefore, simulated experiences can serve as an alternative setting to train surgeons before exposing patients to undue risk.[7] Other factors driving an increased role of simulation in medical education include new techniques and increased procedure and technique complexity, costs and limited access to cadaveric training, a lack of standardized objective assessments of skills, and less instructional time because of work hour restrictions and limited flexibility in faculty schedules.[2,8,9]

EDUCATIONAL TECHNOLOGY IN MEDICAL EDUCATION

The Association for Educational Communications and Technology defines educational technology as the study and ethical practice of facilitating learning and improving performance by creating, using, and managing appropriate technological processes and resources.[10] Thus, educational technology is one aspect of teaching and learning that is meant to create an environment that engages students in the learning process and promotes diverse learning experiences. However, educational technology in medical education more narrowly focuses on devices to deliver and enhance content.[2] Many times this involves using technology developed for clinical practice as an educational tool instead of using technology developed for education. For example, the use of computer-assisted gait analysis to objectively assess lower extremity biomechanics impacts clinical practice, but over time it has impacted podiatric education.

Educational technologies are used to facilitate management of systems, processes, and procedures to aid in task completion. Media and other tools can also assist in accessing content, which is crucial with the vast and constantly changing medical knowledge. Lastly, these tools are used to provide alternative formats for delivering information to optimize students' ability to learn and to retain knowledge. Because it is well known that not everyone learns the same way, this final use of the educational technologies is critical to ensuring all students have opportunities to learn and retain the information necessary to be a successful practitioner.

Online learning is one of the most common types of educational technology impacting medical education. This involves synchronous and asynchronous learning activities, and multimedia for online lectures, virtual patients, and other online communication for feedback and self-assessments. Health information technology is an emerging type of educational technology that can optimize access to information and clinical decision making through real-time processing and sorting information into an organized framework. The significant changes impacting electronic medical records, population health data, and big data systems suggests a more robust role for health information technology as large datasets are used for artificial intelligence and other opportunities to enhance knowledge, support decision making, and quality improvement.[11–13] Educational technology, such as interactive textbooks, digital flashcards, and active learning platforms for real-time class participation and quizzes, enhance student engagement.

Simulation is another key type of technology used in medical education. This involves some hands-on skills training, computerized standardized patients, augmented reality, and VR. Ultimately, simulations move medical education toward a more objective, proficiency-based system, which Pedowitz and Marsh[14] predict will dramatically change surgical skills training. Simulations can also improve patient safety because training occurs in a safe environment where errors are an acceptable part of the learning process. The drivers of simulation-based training in medical education are listed in **Box 1.**

Based on these factors driving the use of simulations, and the evidence showing the significantly enhanced performance of surgical skills in simulation-based trainees compared with conventional methods, simulation-based training will likely expand to longitudinal assessment of medical knowledge and skills.[8] The longitudinal assessment is possible because the simulations can provide knowledge, skills acquisition, and behavioral performance spanning the continuum of medical education, from medical student to provider. For example, continuing education allows providers to reinforce skills, acquire new skills, reenter practice, or meet regulatory needs. Ultimately simulation-based education facilitates medical education competency-based initiatives. The feedback systems in simulation training must incorporate evidence-based knowledge and personal experience.[2] This allows individualization of standardized simulations, which compared with conventional medical education methods, can also improve retention by providing learning environments immersing the learner in emotionally rewarding and dynamic experiences that enhance motivation and provide a sense of achievement.[15]

VIRTUAL REALITY IN MEDICAL EDUCATION

VR in medical education has been a recent development as VR has undergone significant enhancements in quality and capability. However, to be a successful method of teaching, simulations must have construct validity, which distinguishes between experience levels of the user, and concurrent validity, which demonstrates transferability from the simulated setting to the real-world setting.

A systematic review demonstrated improved learning in 74% of studies. More importantly, Samadbeik and colleagues[16] found VR simulations transferred to improved clinical outcomes. They reported 87% higher accuracy in practice, 95% improved skills of trainees, and reduced training time. Other studies also report VR simulations result in improved clinical skills in the OR. Inexperienced residents learning colonoscopy and endoscopy using VR had lower performance errors and greater accuracy compared with those who trained conventionally through learning via direct

---

Box 1
The factors driving the use of simulation-based training in medical education

- The need for an objective, proficiency-based system (competency-based education).
- Enhance educational efficiency through structured curriculum and objective, standardized assessments.
- Training occurs in safe environment optimizing patient safety.
- Improves limited patient availability occurring with shortages of clinical training sites.
- Improves limited exposure to rare conditions.
- Improves limited access to cadaveric training.
- Improves training of new and more complex techniques.
- Can be more cost-effective method training.
- Makes training more accessible despite decreased instructional time caused by work hour restrictions and limited flexibility in faculty schedules.

Data from Refs.[2,8,9,14]

patient care.[17–19] **Box 2** displays a general list of advantages and disadvantages of VR simulation in medical education.

Most of the literature investigates uses of VR developed for post-graduate medical education. Effective VR simulations have been develop for medical resident training in invasive hemodynamic monitoring, mechanical ventilation, and standardized educational intervention.[16] Moreover, Schroedl and colleagues[20] reported VR simulation improved the knowledge and skills of residents in the intensive care unit. The authors concluded VR simulation is an invaluable approach for standard medical education.

Post-graduate surgical specialties dominate the implementation of VR-based education. Laparoscopic surgery and orthopedic surgery have studied the use VR in training residents the most, although other surgical specialties integrate VR into their post-graduate programs. The more basic uses teach suturing and knot tying, which has been shown to improve the speed and mobility of practitioners in the OR.[21] Multiple studies demonstrate the concurrent validity of the skills integrated in laparoscopic simulations.[22–24] Studies using an endoscopic sinus surgery VR simulator found surgeons trained to proficiency with established criteria were equivalent or outperformed conventionally trained participants.[25]

One of the more simplistic uses in orthopedic surgery provides fracture anatomy instruction.[26] Meanwhile training in bone cuts using VR simulation has proven to be a safe, cost-effective, and repeatable method of instruction for beginning and experienced orthopedic surgeons because the simulations helped improve their recognition skill of anatomic positions.[27] Studies of knee and shoulder arthroscopy demonstrate improvement in performance of skills with repeated use, whereas other studies demonstrate the ability to distinguish the users experience level and the progression along the competency learning curve. However, orthopedic VR simulations of other procedures lack evidence of concurrent validity.[7]

Despite the new generation of digital native learners who expect and are accustomed to technology-enhanced learning environments, medical students have only recently been exposed to VR-based video segments of simulations demonstrating palliative and end-of-life care and anatomy and neuroanatomy VR simulations. These simulations have proven to be effective with all of them reporting increased immersion, motivation, and engagement in the learning process.[28–30] The neuroanatomy simulations also observed improved retention.[28]

Box 2
Advantages and disadvantages of virtual reality simulation in medical education

Advantages	Disadvantages
• Increased student engagement, motivation, and self-confidence	• Cost of VR simulator development, equipment, and implementation
• Enhanced understanding of 3-dimensional anatomy and relationships between anatomic structures	• Adjunctive, not a replacement for real experience
• Improved retention	• Not truly self-learning, faculty feedback is required to optimize benefits of simulation-based training
• Increased skills	• Currently limited availability, especially for medical students
• Reduced time to acquire competency	• Haptic technology for tactile feedback during simulation still lacking and requires data from live surgery to configure sensors to provide realistic feedback during simulation
• Improved patient safety	
• Improved accuracy, reduced errors in surgical skills	

Although VR simulations are considered a beneficial component of medical education, it is widely regarded to be an adjunctive component of the curriculum delivery, not serving to replace traditional training. Therefore, students must experience real-world patient care, yet simulation can advance training without exposing patients to untrained providers. Ultimately this augments the medical education mantra of "see one, do one, teach one," which is wrought with performance and ethical dilemmas, by advancing the surgical learning curve before direct patient care.[31]

THE WESTERN UNIVERSITY COLLEGE OF PODIATRIC MEDICINE VIRTUAL OPERATING ROOM

The WesternU CPM is developing a VR OR suite (**Fig. 1**). The WesternU virtual OR is a unique use of educational technology because it brings virtual surgical skills training to students before residency training and it is the first use of VR simulations designed specifically for podiatric medical education. The design of the virtual OR for podiatric education addresses the specific needs of one of the few fields of medicine that undergoes specialty-specific training before their residency. Developing simulations specific to podiatric surgery aligns with a systematic review on the application of VR simulation in medical group education that concluded VR simulations specific to the needs of the group is an appropriate solution for effective training.[16]

Although achieving success using VR simulations relies on improved learning that translates to improved clinical outcomes, students gain valuable lessons by first learning the general rules and how to function in the OR, the instrumentation, and basic surgical skills. The design of the WesternU virtual OR allows students to gain this knowledge before entering the real-world OR. Our goals listed in **Box 3** are multifaceted.

With these goals in mind, WesternU virtual OR instructional design teaches the principles and knowledge surrounding basic functioning in an OR through performing surgical procedures in a stepwise approach. The first module developed was designed to teach students instrumentation most applicable to the podiatric surgeon. The goal of this module is to instruct students on the basic function indication of each instrument. The next module provides instruction in gowning, gloving, and sterile technique, followed by modules on incision placement and suturing and knot tying. In the fifth module students perform basic foot and ankle surgery. This provides students a gradual progression of the content as they are introduced to the OR, which slowly increases their responsibilities as they gain understanding, proficiency, and eventually mastery of the required knowledge and skills.

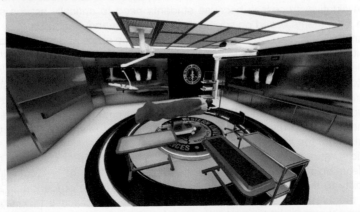

Fig. 1. The WesternU virtual operating room. (Courtesy of WesternU Department of Podiatric Medicine, Surgery and Biomechanics, Pomona, CA.)

Box 3
Goals of the WesternU virtual operating room

- Improve the learning experience by reducing anxiety associated with initial exposure to the real-world environment, allowing students to focus on what and why something is done, instead of being overwhelmed.

- Engage students in the learning process, to improve their appreciation, understanding, and retention.

- Improve patient safety by improving students' skills without the undue risk of providing patient care during the initial learning experience.

- Facilitate the development of competency-based education by assessing student knowledge, ability to perform surgical skills, and appropriate behaviors at an acceptable level for podiatric medical students.

OR teams are a prime example of the interprofessional teams Han and colleagues[2] claim can benefit from simulation technology because of the inherent complexity of OR teams, competencies of multiple providers, and the health care system. Additional virtual OR modules being developed focus on the World Health Organization "Time-out" to focus on team communication skills and patient safety, followed by a module on team functions to address intraoperative complications. Students will train on interprofessional teams involving osteopathic and nursing students on completion of the podiatric surgical modules. This experience will help teach our students how to function on complex, multidisciplinary teams by enhancing communication skills and professionalism. This maximizes the true benefit of simulations, by teaching how to protect patients before having to protect them. In addition, this creates a more active VR experience compared with the current VR uses in medical education.

Each module begins providing content by using the simulation tool to improving access to information, so students learn factual and conceptual knowledge. As students progress through each module, the complexity of the knowledge and cognition increases. Students move from the more basic cognition types of factual and conceptual cognition to procedural cognition in most modules. The interprofessional team-based modules require metacognitive knowledge, which is the most advanced type of cognition. All of the modules begin with remembering and understanding, which are the two lowest levels of learning. The podiatric modules progress to analyzing and applying the knowledge learned, whereas the multidisciplinary teams-based modules elevate reliance on evaluative processes because students need to critically assess situations and make judgements based on specific learned criteria and standards.

For example, as students handle the instruments, the name and indications of each instrument are displayed on the virtual OR anesthesia monitors (**Figs. 2** and **3**). Once students learn the instruments, they begin the second phase of the module, requiring students to identify instruments to set up for a given procedure, where the instruments needed are listed on the monitors. The final phase of the module is an assessment, where students apply their knowledge of surgical instruments by setting up the stand without the list of instruments, requiring them to process the steps of the surgery and the indications of the instruments.

Podiatric surgery residents reported immediate feedback after surgery is the most valuable learning resource.[32] When using simulators, a lack of feedback limits the transferability to the real world.[33] To address the importance of feedback, students complete modules with a classmate present so they can discuss their experience and reinforce the material learned immediately following the simulation. In addition, clinical faculty review the assessments integrated within the simulation and provide

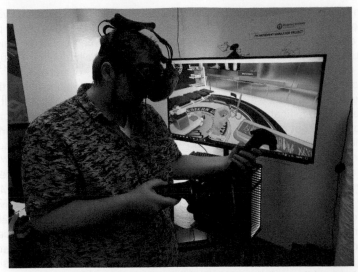

Fig. 2. A student using the WesternU virtual operating room. (Courtesy of WesternU Department of Podiatric Medicine, Surgery and Biomechanics, Pomona, CA.)

timely feedback via face-to-face discussions. Students are also asked to complete a questionnaire about their experience to improve simulations and to gain valuable feedback regarding the role of VR as an engaging method of delivering and assessing student competency.

To study the benefits of the virtual OR as a novel educational technology tool integrated in the clinical education curriculum, we designed a study to test our hypothesis that virtual OR simulations are an engaging method of delivering and assessing surgical knowledge and skills of podiatric medical students that aids retention and reduces anxiety normally experienced when first exposed to the real-world OR.

MATERIALS AND METHODS

Surveys will be sent to students to assess their perception of the surgical instrument content delivery using the virtual OR compared with the conventional method. The

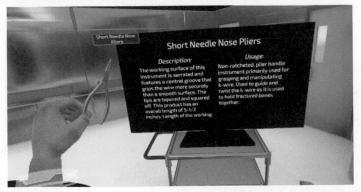

Fig. 3. The first module of the WesternU virtual operating involves handling instruments while learning about the instrument and its indications. (Courtesy of WesternU Department of Podiatric Medicine, Surgery and Biomechanics, Pomona, CA.)

study was approved by the WesternU International Review Board. Students voluntarily participate in the anonymous survey administered using a cloud-based survey platform.

Before administering surveys, students receive an informed consent, which mentions the uncommon and transient risks associated with VR simulations, including difficulty or discomfort with glasses and headset, dizziness, or vertigo.[30,34] Another student accompanies each participant immersed in the VR simulation during the entire session, which helps reduce the potential risk of falls or other injury as a result of dizziness or vertigo. To mitigate students perceiving a potentially negative impact on their grade should they not complete the survey, the informed consent also clearly states participation is voluntary and that incomplete surveys or no response has no impact on their grade.

Survey administration uses purposive sampling, a nonrandom selection technique for survey administration to capture members of a specific population.[35] CPM classes 2019 and 2020 serve as the control group because they experienced conventional methods of delivering the surgical instrumentation content. CPM classes 2021 and 2022 will receive surveys assessing the virtual OR. The study group will receive surveys on completing the first VR module and after completing their first podiatric rotation during the clinical curriculum. Data are stored in Qualtrics and the analysis will be performed using Microsoft Excel/Word (Seattle, WA).

Survey results will be compared using descriptive statistics. The significance between groups (defined as $P<.05$) will be assessed using Student t-test and chi-square test for continuous and categorical variables, respectively. Transferability of the knowledge and skills learned in the simulations will be assessed using podiatric physician clinical evaluations. Future assessment of the virtual OR includes skills performance accuracy using assessments integrated within future modules.

SUMMARY

Dan Schulman, CEO of PayPal, has said, "The biggest impediment to a company's future success is its past success." Accepting and adopting the role of educational technology is key to moving medical education forward. To truly reap the benefits requires changing how we manage curriculum, from enrollment to content delivery to monitoring and tracking assessments. At WesternU we are launching a virtual OR to deliver surgical training from instrumentation to preforming procedures and interprofessional education. This provides students a novel method of instruction that addresses generational learning needs and limitations in medical education. In addition, this innovative tool affords students experiences that potentially enhance skills and retention with less anxiety that comes with initial exposure to the OR, which can lead to a downstream benefit of improved patient safety.

DISCLOSURE

The authors have nothing to disclose.

REFERENCES

1. Engel CE. Educational technology in medical education. Proc R Soc Med 1972; 65:771–3.
2. Han H, Resch DS, Kovach RA. Educational technology in medical education. Teach Learn Med 2013;25(S1):S39–43.
3. McGaghie WC, Issenberg SB, Cohen ER, et al. Does simulation based-medical education with deliberate practice yield better results than traditional clinical

education? A meta-analytic comparative review of the evidence. Acad Med 2011; 86:706–11.

4. Zendejas B, Brydges R. Patient outcomes in simulation-based medical education: a systematic review. J Gen Intern Med 2013;28:1078–89.

5. Densen P. Challenges and opportunities facing medical education. Trans Am Clin Climatol Assoc 2011;122:48–58.

6. Guze PA. Using technology to meet the challenges of medical education. Trans Am Clin Climatol Assoc 2015;126:260–70.

7. Bartlett JD, Lawrence JE, Stewart ME. Instructional review: does virtual reality simulation have a role in training trauma and orthopaedic surgeons? J Bone Joint Surg 2018;100-B(5):559–65.

8. Atesok K, Satava RM, Van Hest A, et al. Retention of skills after simulation-based training in orthopaedic surgery. J Am Acad Orthop Surg 2016;24(8):505–14.

9. Gardner AK, Scott DJ, Pedowitz RA, et al. Best practices across surgical specialties relating to simulation-based training. Surgery 2015;158(5):1395–402.

10. Januszewski A, Persichitte KA. A history of the AECT's definitions of educational technology. In: Zanuszewski A, Molenda M, editors. Educational technology: a definition with commentary. New York: Taylor & Francis; 2008. p. 259–82.

11. Barnett GO. Information technology and medical education. J Am Med Inform Assoc 1995;2:285–91.

12. Hammond MM, Margo K, Christner JG, et al. Opportunities and challenges in integrating electronic health records into undergraduate medical education: a national survey of clerkship directors. Teach Learn Med 2012;24:219–24.

13. Spencer DC, Choi D, English C, et al. The effects of electronic health record implementation on medical student educators. Teach Learn Med 2012;24:106–10.

14. Pedowitz RA, Marsh JL. Motor skills training in orthopaedic surgery: a paradigm shift toward simulation-based educational curriculum. J Am Acad Orthop Surg 2012;20(7):407–9.

15. Dale E. Audiovisual methods in teaching. New York: Dryden Press; 1969.

16. Samadbeik M, Yaaghobi D, Bastani P, et al. The applications of virtual reality technology on medical groups teaching. J Adv Med Educ Prof 2018;6(3):123–9.

17. Eversbusch A, Grantcharov TP. Learning curves and impact of psychomotor training on performance in simulated colonoscopy: a randomized trial using a virtual reality endoscopy trainer. Surg Endosc 2004;18:1514–8.

18. Felsher JJ, Olesevich M, Farres H, et al. Validation of a flexible endoscopy simulator. Am J Surg 2005;189:497–500.

19. Grantcharov TP, Carstensen L, Schulze S. Objective assessment of gastrointestinal endoscopy skills using a virtual reality simulator. JSLS 2005;9:130–3.

20. Schroedl CJ, Corbridge TC, Cohen ER, et al. Use of simulation-based education to improve resident learning and patient care in the medical intensive care unit: a randomized trial. J Crit Care 2012;27(2):219.

21. Yoganathan S, Finch DA, Parkin E, et al. 360° virtual reality video for the acquisition of knot tying skills: a randomized controlled trial. Int J Surg 2018;54:24–7.

22. Alaker M, Wynn GR, Arulampalam T. Virtual reality training in laparoscopic surgery: a systematic review and meta-analysis. Int J Surg 2016;29:85–94.

23. Korndorffer JR, Dunne JB, Sierra R, et al. Simulator training for laparoscopic suturing using performance goals translates to the operating room. J Am Coll Surg 2005;201:23–9.

24. Seymour NE, Gallagher AG, Roman SA, et al. Virtual reality training improves operating room performance: results of a randomized, double-blinded study. Ann Surg 2002;236:458–63.

25. Fried MP, Sadoughi B, Gibber MJ, et al. From virtual reality to the operating room: the endoscopic sinus surgery simulator experiment. Otolaryngol Head Neck Surg 2010;142:202–7.

26. Bongers PJ, Van Hove PD, Stassen LP, et al. A new virtual-reality training module for laparoscopic surgical skills and equipment handling: can multitasking be trained? A randomized controlled trial. J Surg Educ 2015;72(2):184–91.

27. Lin Y, Wang X, Wu F, et al. Development and validation of a surgical training simulator with haptic feedback for learning bone-sawing skill. J Biomed Inform 2014; 48:122–9.

28. Ekstrand C, Jamal A, Nguyen R, et al. Immersive and interactive virtual reality to improve learning and retention in neuroanatomy in medical students: a randomized controlled study. CMAJ Open 2018;6(10):E103–9.

29. Moro C, Stromberga Z, Raikos A, et al. The effectiveness of virtual and augmented reality in health sciences and medical anatomy. Anat Sci Educ 2017;10:549–59.

30. Taubert M, Webber L, Hamilton T, et al. Virtual reality videos used in undergraduate palliative and oncology medical teaching: results of a pilot study. BMJ Support Palliat Care 2019;9(3):281–5.

31. Pedowitz R. Commentary & perspective. Moving from "see one, do one, teach one": simulation training can save money. J Bone Joint Surg 2017;99A:e97(1-2).

32. Shofler D, Chuang T, Argade N. The residency training experience in podiatric medicine and surgery. J Foot Ankle Surg 2015;54(4):607–14.

33. Oestergaard J, Bjerrum F, Maagaard M, et al. Instructor feedback versus no instructor feedback on performance in a laparoscopic virtual reality simulator: a randomized educational trial. BMC Med Educ 2012;12:7.

34. Wang Q, Li C, Xie Z, et al. The development and application of virtual reality animation simulation technology: take gastroscopy simulation system as an example. Pathol Oncol Res 2019. https://doi.org/10.1007/s12253-019-00590-8.

35. Kelley K, Clark B, Brown V, et al. Good practice in the conduct and reporting of survey research. Int J Qual Health Care 2003;15(3):261–6.

Moving?

Make sure your subscription moves with you!

To notify us of your new address, find your **Clinics Account Number** (located on your mailing label above your name), and contact customer service at:

Email: journalscustomerservice-usa@elsevier.com

800-654-2452 (subscribers in the U.S. & Canada)
314-447-8871 (subscribers outside of the U.S. & Canada)

Fax number: 314-447-8029

Elsevier Health Sciences Division
Subscription Customer Service
3251 Riverport Lane
Maryland Heights, MO 63043

*To ensure uninterrupted delivery of your subscription, please notify us at least 4 weeks in advance of move.

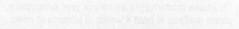

Printed and bound by CPI Group (UK) Ltd, Croydon, CR0 4YY

03/10/2024

01040484-0010